Special Praise for *Game P...*

"*Game Plan* was created and enriched by three distinct but deeply aligned sensibilities, each seasoned by experience and blessed with compassion. The book that has resulted from this synthesis is both rich and concise, both practical and inspirational. Those who read and apply it will be well informed and prepared to go forward with hope and purpose."

Archie Brodsky
Department of Psychiatry
Beth Israel Deaconess Medical Center,
Harvard Medical School
Coauthor of *Love and Addiction* and
The Truth About Addiction and Recovery

"It seems that a book on men's emotional fitness would have a very specific and narrow audience. But it actually has lots of information, insights, and practical help for men, women, counselors, therapists, other helping professionals, and programs. If you are a man and are considering this book, you are well on your way to getting the full benefit of the exploration and exercises inside these pages. If you are a woman, be prepared to understand and accept the men in your life much better. If you are a helping professional, there's a lot here that you were never taught and need to know."

David Mee-Lee, MD
Psychiatrist and Addiction Specialist
DML Training and Consulting
Davis, California

"*Game Plan* is a valuable contribution to the sparse literature for and about men. It provides helpful insights about the forces in today's society that shape men's lives. The exercises and tools within its pages lead the reader through an exploration of the 'big' issues, such as sexuality, emotion, addiction, and money. This is an essential resource for men, those who live with them, and especially those who counsel them."

Michael Hoge, PhD
Professor of Psychiatry
Yale School of Medicine

"This book achieves two important functions. It will help both professional helpers and clients do their jobs. It is an excellent resource for professionals who are in need of information and a set of readily applicable tools. My male clients will find it helpful in their pursuit of personal growth. I will certainly use it extensively for my clients and will add it to the bibliotherapy list I give them. Thank you for this invaluable tool."

William L. Mock, PhD, LISW, LICDC, SAP
Executive Director, Center for Interpersonal
Development, Ohio

"*Game Plan* has been a wonderful tool in my private practice toolbox, both for me as a practitioner and for my clients. The authors recognize the attractive and not-so-attractive parts of themselves through the stories and exercises presented in this book."

Rachel Green, PhD
Psychologist, Motivational Interviewing
Trainer, and Founder of Dancing Gecko
Training, Montreal, Québec

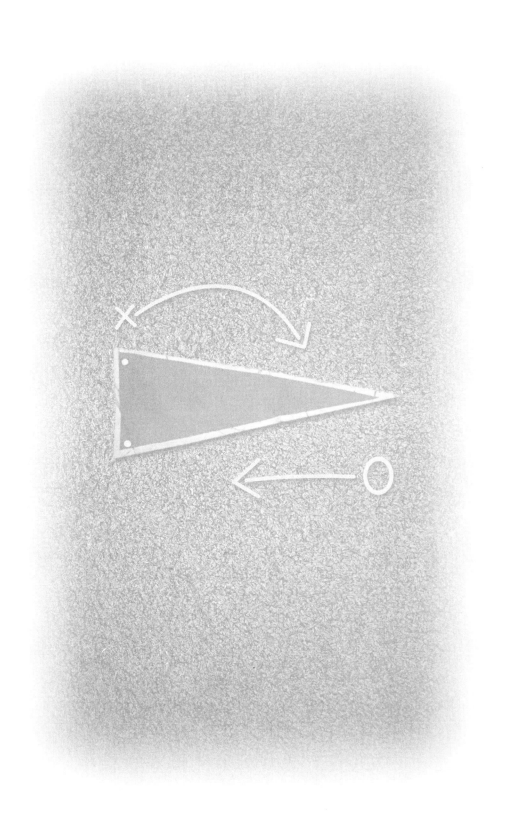

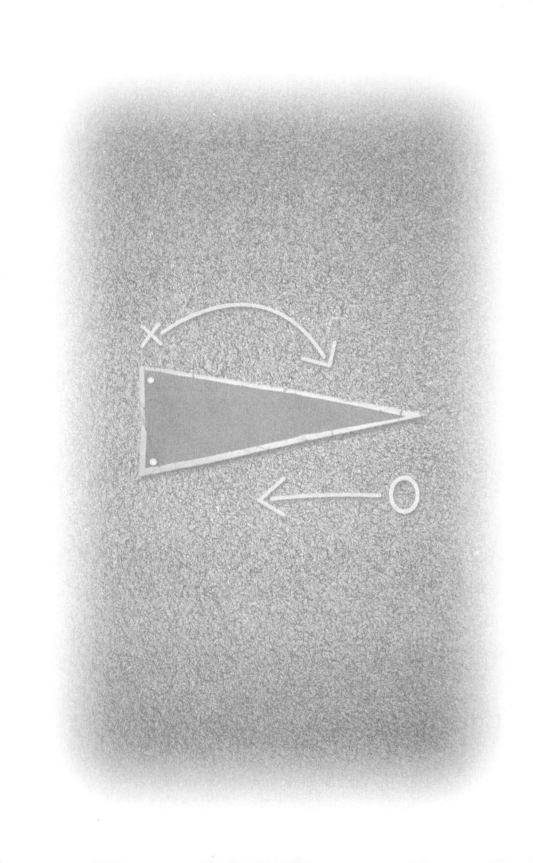

Game Plan

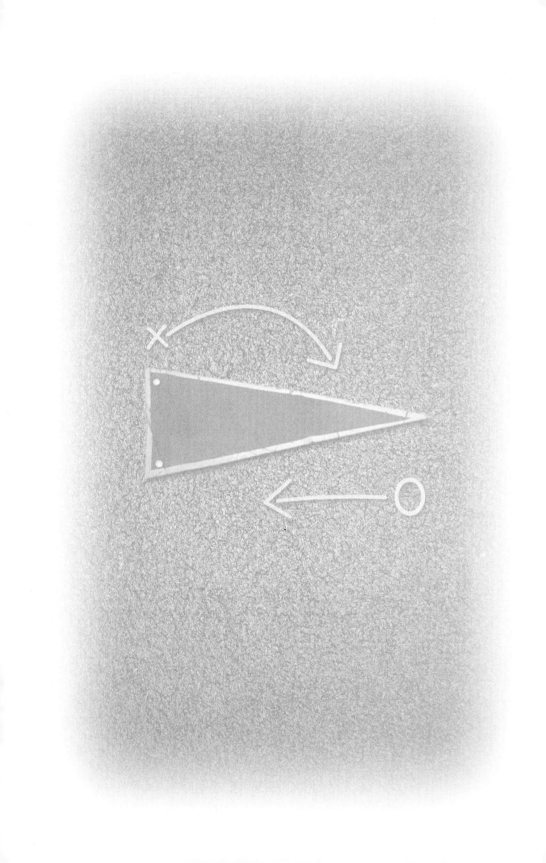

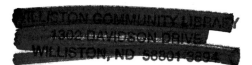

Game Plan

A Man's Guide to Achieving Emotional Fitness

Alan P. Lyme, David J. Powell,
and Stephen R. Andrew

CENTRAL RECOVERY PRESS

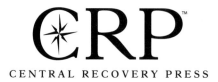

CENTRAL RECOVERY PRESS

Central Recovery Press (CRP) is committed to publishing exceptional materials addressing addiction treatment, recovery, and behavioral healthcare, including original and quality books, audio/visual communications, and web-based new media. Through a diverse selection of titles, we seek to contribute to a broad range of unique resources for professionals, recovering individuals and their families, and the general public.

For more information, visit **www.centralrecoverypress.com**

Central Recovery Press, Las Vegas, NV 89129

Publisher: Central Recovery Press
             3321 N. Buffalo Drive
             Las Vegas, NV 89129

17 16 15 14 13 12   1 2 3 4 5

ISBN-13: 978-1-936290-96-3 (paper)
ISBN-13: 978-1-937612-04-7 (e-book)

Photo of David Powell © Tom Croke/Visual Image, Inc. Used with permission. Photo of Alan Lyme © John Knight. Used with permission. Photo of Stephen Andrew © Richard G. Sandifer. Used with permission.

Publisher's Note: This book contains general information about addiction and other self-destructive behaviors, and developing wellness and emotional health. The information is not medical advice, and should not be treated as such. Central Recovery Press makes no representations or warranties in relation to any medical information in this book; this book is not an alternative to medical advice from your doctor or other professional healthcare provider. If you have any specific questions about any medical matter you should consult your doctor or other professional healthcare provider. If you think you or someone close to you may be suffering from any medical or mental health condition, you should seek immediate medical attention. You should never delay seeking medical advice, disregard medical advice, or discontinue medical treatment because of information in this or any book.

Our books represent the experiences and opinions of their authors only. Every effort has been made to ensure that events, institutions, and statistics presented in our books as facts are accurate and up-to-date. To protect their privacy, some of the names of people and institutions have been changed.

Book design by David Leicester Hardy

Table of Contents

Section III: Helping Men/Healing Men

Section IV: Resources for Healing

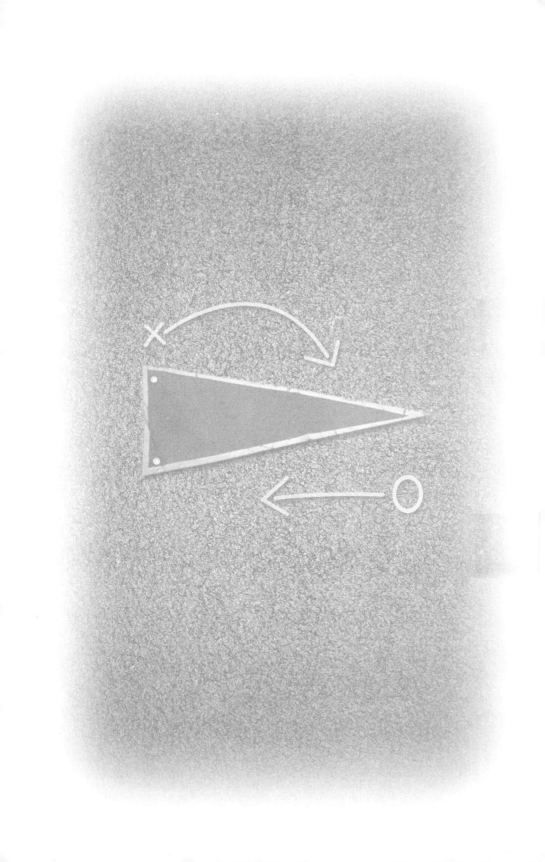

Foreword

For nearly twenty-five years, I've been working on my own "men's issues," and have counseled, coached, and facilitated men's groups, workshops, and conferences. I've read virtually every book written for and about men and have even written a few of my own. I've been taught by and have had the privilege to teach with leaders in men's work—greats like Robert Bly, Dr. Robert Moore, Malidoma Somé, Robert Johnson, and several others.

So when my friend Alan Lyme sent me *Game Plan* and asked me to read it and write the foreword, I was a little reluctant to read yet another "men's book." Man, was I pleasantly surprised and delighted! I found myself underlining all kinds of things I'd never heard said or had never thought of before. The authors of *Game Plan*—Alan Lyme, David J. Powell, and Stephen Andrew—are brilliant, powerful men. They not only have put their hearts, heads, and souls into this book, but also have included genuinely useful tools to help anyone who loves, lives with, or works with men. Thanks to books like this one, men, women, and children will be forever different than my generation and previous generations.

For instance, your teenage son just broke up with his first girlfriend. He tells his buddies about it, and here's what is so different from previous generations of men: he feels absolutely free to ask for support to get over it. He even sheds a few tears, but not one of his friends makes fun of him or calls him names. His masculinity is never called into question. How did this happen?

Your stressed-out husband opens up and tells you how scared he is in the down economy and you don't think he is weak or inferior in any way. You are not nearly as worried as you would be if he kept all his feelings buried or bottled up like your father and grandfather were taught to do. How did this come about?

Your boss is interested in all his employees' well-being and has even been described as a man who puts people before profits. Many have commented that he is a man who really listens and cares.

Your youngest nephew is often paraded out as a man who does not hesitate to nurture his new baby and takes a leave of absence from his job to do so.

Remember the day when two gay men could not adopt, and certainly no primetime television show would dare show it?

How in the hell did this transformation from men like Don Draper of *Mad Men* to men like Dr. McDreamy from *Grey's Anatomy* happen?

Read *Game Plan* and you will have a good many answers.

There is a new man in town—in our homes, in office buildings and factories, in the Speaker of the House chair, and behind the desk in the Oval Office. He makes regular appearances on the big and small screens and on the Internet. This is a man who has benefited from the kind of material that can be found in *Game Plan*. He and his sons have been given a full pass to be as emotionally expressive and expansive as their wives, daughters, or mothers have always been. Where did this new man come from? Who brought about this sea change? Men like the ones who wrote this wonderful book.

We all have heard about the feminist movement and what it achieved. Everyone knows what a huge impact the civil rights movement has had on society. Both movements made us more conscious human beings and worked toward leveling the economic and political playing fields. But what about this thing called the men's movement? The role this movement played in changing the status quo, redefining masculinity, and freeing men in a multitude of ways affects nearly every facet of daily life. Yes, there really was a game plan, though many of us didn't know it at the time, and its legacy is now a set of norms we take for granted.

How things have changed.

The authors of *Game Plan* have achieved three important things extremely well:

1. They have brought their collective knowledge, wisdom, and years of experience in working with men and put it into one manual.

2. They have successfully pulled together the best ideas, insights, information, and guidance from their own mentors and teachers into a single, powerful book.

3. They have written it all down in a highly organized and reader-friendly way.

To be a man in these ever-changing times is challenging to say the least. Speaking for myself, I need all the help I can get to navigate my whitewater ride through work, relationships, recovery, parenting, and friendship. I received some real guidance from reading this book, and I know you will as well.

There is an old Arabic proverb that says, "A man sets out on a journey that takes him two hundred years to complete. If he had a good guide it would have only taken him two days." With this book, you have a good guide, a toolbox full of important information, and three mentors who are a step or two further along on this journey into deep manhood and recovery. I hope you read it, do the very powerful exercises in it, ponder its wisdom, and pass it on.

John Lee
Author of *The Flying Boy* and *The Half-Lived Life*

Author's Note

This manual began as a germ of an idea between David Powell, Stephen Andrew, and me, Alan Lyme. It was originally intended to be a small workbook to be used by the residents in a men's treatment facility in West Palm Beach, Florida. With the addition of the prolific David Powell, the work grew in size and scope and began to take on a life of its own. It became apparent that the manual might be of some use to a larger audience, with something for everyone. Thus was born the first manifestation of this work, known as *Men's Healing: A Toolbox for Life*. In the years since that publication, much changed for the authors and indeed for men all across the country. Jobs came and went, families shifted and grew, and friendships were developed and lost. *Game Plan* is our attempt to update the work we began in 2006, revisiting some of the ideas and stories through the new lens of our collective experience.

I'd like to thank John Lee for his thoughtful foreword and continued support. He speaks of mentors, and I have been blessed with this opportunity to collaborate with mine.

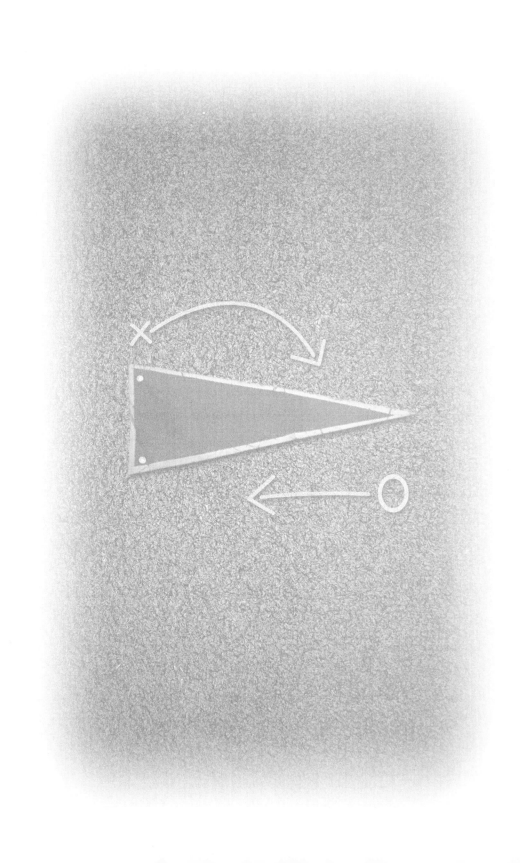

Introduction

Real men don't ask for help! Early in our development, we are taught to take care of ourselves, to do it ourselves, to not ask for help. Yet most men come to a fork in life's road that requires them to change direction. This could be the result of aging and maturing, illness, lifestyle changes, addiction, loss of employment, significant relationships, or other life stressors. Whatever the cause, our tendency to "do it ourselves" no longer works and we need to find new tools to deal with life's ever-changing course.

What is needed is a practical manual that discusses how men can get help and how to help men. The goal of this manual is twofold: to give care providers of men the tools they need to help men heal, and to offer to men a guide for self-discovery.

Johnny Carson, the comedian, would say, "When you come to the fork in the road, take it." But what direction should we take at the fork? This "game plan" for men offers knowledge and skills to be used throughout life, and especially when faced with significant life changes.

The hypothesis of this manual is that men do well when working with other men. There are several qualities that most men have in common: a sense of competition and comparison; an action-oriented, problem-solving style when dealing with life issues; a clear sense of the "rules" in playing the game of life (which are often learned through sports); and, currently, some degree of confusion about what it means to be a man in a world where gender roles are rapidly changing.

This is a game plan for men's lives, Version 2.0. Version 1.0 was entitled *Men's Healing: A Toolbox for Life*, and was germinated in the fertile soil of a residential gender-specific and age-appropriate treatment program for both those afflicted with addiction and the dually diagnosed. It was there that the authors came together and began to explore the concept of a joint writing venture. Alan Lyme was program director at that treatment center and had consulted with Stephen Andrew of the Health and Education Training Institute of Portland, Maine on both gender-specific treatment for men and the campus-wide training on Motivational Interviewing. Stephen, in turn, introduced David Powell, president of the International Center for Health Concerns, Inc. David, who had spent his career as an author, clinician, and clinical supervisor, began a consultant relationship with the center on both working with men and clinical supervision.

Version 1.0 was a collaboration among these three men who had a similar vision. That vision included freeing men from the bondage of their collective past and helping them to create a limitless future. We no longer have to pretend to be GI Joe, the Marlboro Man, or a superhero. We do not have to perpetuate our fathers' addiction to work, alcohol, or emotional obscurity. We can feel, love, trust, and be vulnerable. All of the material contained within the first version of the book was "field-tested" with the male clients at Hanley Center, and the results were very encouraging.

Since Version 1.0 was published in 2008, each of us has gone through some significant life changes ourselves. Version 2.0 reflects the lessons we have learned as we moved through these changes.

Alan Lyme left Florida and is now working in Macon, Georgia as a clinical supervisor for a Substance Abuse and Mental Health Services Administration (SAMHSA) research project. He continues to teach Motivational Interviewing, skills for working with men, and clinical supervision to a national audience. He remarried, is the proud father of his first son, and has settled into a new life in rural Georgia.

David Powell has moved to semiretirement (or as he calls it, "refirement") and is learning through trial and error a new word— "no"—and how to say it. After thirty-two years of working in China, he has turned that effort over to younger Turks to carry the work into the next generation.

Stephen Andrew's family moved to London to try out "being British," and recently returned to living together in Portland, Maine, where Stephen continues his work at the Health Education and Training Institute. He also continues to teach Motivational Interviewing to people working in criminal justice and healthcare, and loves to bring compassion into everyday care conversations. These life changes have brought new challenges and perspective to each of us. Version 2.0 is an attempt to share our new insights.

Game Plan is written for both the general reader and care providers. The first half of the book offers an explanation of the most important issues facing men today and provides the necessary tools for the average man to work through them. The second half of the book offers care providers ideas about how to help their male care receivers address these issues. This section reviews strategies for working with men, helpful modules for psychoeducation, Motivational Interviewing skills when counseling men, and key issues to address in caregiving. The book then presents practical techniques for the care provider, including exercises and activities to use, rites and rituals to perform to help men through the passage into a recovery-oriented manhood.

Although written with the care provider in mind, the second section is also a great source of information for anyone seeking a deeper understanding of the man's journey.

There are several major themes that are important to men's work, which run throughout the book. These themes are:

- Maintaining hope
- Establishing healthy communication
- Dealing with isolation and violence
- Transforming pain
- Overcoming shame and moving toward humility and acceptance
- Stopping chronic negative thinking
- Living in the here and now, being fully present

The case studies in the book are composites of a number of men whom we have been blessed to work with. They are included to illuminate the vast experience and hope of those who have had the courage to challenge their life path. All names and identifying information have been changed to maintain anonymity and confidentiality.

Throughout the book, we use the word "care provider" as a generic term encompassing a variety of individuals working with men: counselors, spiritual guides, mentors, psychotherapists, life coaches, medical personnel, social workers, family counselors, etc. When appropriate, we will refer specifically to counselors, and more specifically, professionals who treat those who abuse alcohol and other drugs.

Because the book is written by men, primarily for men, we use the masculine gender. We hope that women will feel equally welcome to take advantage of whatever information they deem pertinent.

In the recent history of publishing, the majority of the books about men are actually purchased by women. "Look, honey, I bought you a book about men. I read it and highlighted the parts you need to read." This book is meant to be accessible for men and women together, as well as for individuals seeking to better understand the lives of men.

How to Use This Book

At the end of each chapter of this book are helpful hints and summaries for care providers and for men (and women) in general. Active engagement with the material in *Game Plan* is the key to maximum benefit. Simply reading through the issues may be interesting, but will change little unless you seriously consider and apply the information and exercises to your life. Change is not simply a mental activity; rather, it requires a shift in attitude as well as behavior to incorporate these tools into your daily life.

Ultimately, this is a spiritual book, asking questions not only about how to live but also about why we live. It encourages the reader to explore his spirit and the fundamental questions about what it means to be a man in today's ever-changing world.

The exercises throughout the book are designed to be completed in a separate journal, either by the person using the book or as assigned by a care provider to a client as a therapeutic tool to be completed on his own. Keeping a journal enables the reader to apply the perspectives in this book to his specific journey in life. Our hope is that care providers choose to complete the exercises themselves, when appropriate, before assigning them to clients, so as to explore their own personal, emotional, and spiritual histories, and to better understand their clients' explorations. We took into consideration that some (most) care providers using this book to work with men will be women, and we hope that the information contained herein may make their task a little easier.

The book will also provide the reader with the following benefits:

- A new vision of what it is like to be a man today

- Strategies for dealing with challenges men face

- Guidance to answer the basic questions in life, such as, "What's it all about?" and "What is my life's meaning and purpose?"

- Tools to address areas such as addiction, coping with emotions, relationships, sexuality, money, employment, retirement, and barriers to being a wise, giving, and fulfilled man

- Resources to work through key issues in life, including exercises, reading, videos, poetry, art, activities, and questionnaires

- An extensive, updated bibliography related to men's issues

As you read this book, we encourage you to engage in these activities and answer the questions posed, seeking wisdom and not knowledge, insight and not data, and learning to live with life's unanswerable questions.

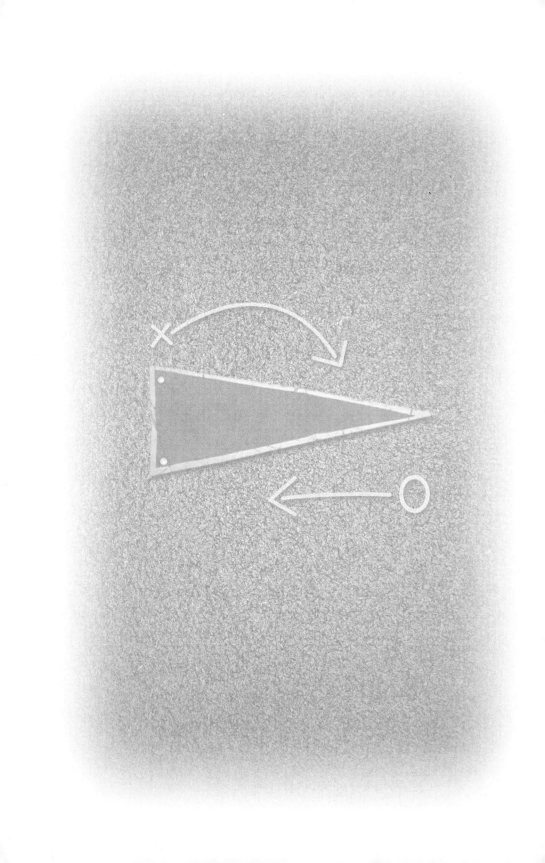

Section I: Being a Man

One: An Environment of Risk

What does it mean to be a man in the twenty-first century? To be a man in this millennium is to be in isolation. We are taught to be in competition with each other and to trust no one. We are expected to be sensitive to the needs of others. We are expected to provide for our families. How do we cope? Many cope by leading meaningless lives of desperation. Food, work, exercise, alcohol and other drugs, sex, sports, spending, religion, pornography, television, and the Internet are some of the ways we cope by avoiding the reality of our existence. Some men are fortunate enough to find support among their peers through social gatherings, church groups, or support groups. But for the majority, isolation is the key habit. When we isolate, we shelter ourselves from feeling. We cloak our emotions with superficiality—smile for the camera called life. Research on men's issues yields the following data for the US population:

- The majority of children abused, neglected, and murdered are boys.[1]

- Most of the children in foster care, shelters, and juvenile institutions are boys.[2]

- Seventy-five percent of student suspensions, expulsions, grade failures, and special education referrals go to boys, and school violence casualties and all other assault victims are included in this number.[3]

- Seventy-nine percent of suicides are boys/men.[4]

- Seventy-five percent of teenage suicides are boys.[5]

- For gay men, the rate of suicide is 1.5 to 2.5 times greater than for heterosexual men.[6]

- Seventy-two percent of the homeless are boys/men.[7]

- Ninety-three percent of prison inmates are men.[8]

- Ninety-nine percent of executed prisoners are men (since 1976, 1,264 men and 12 women).[9]

Looking at these statistics compelled us to examine the underlying causes, as well as the ways every man—especially those in the grip of addiction and other life problems—is affected by those causes. Within moments of being born, males are often treated with less affection than females. Studies have shown that a newborn baby covered with a blue blanket will get touched less and will be spoken to in a firmer voice than the same baby in a pink blanket.[10] Gender-stereotyping behavior on the part of adults, even those sensitive to gender issues, is endemic. This sets the stage for induction into the "boy code," in which emotions need to be kept in check, violence is an acceptable response to emotional upset, self-esteem relies on power, and all "feminine" qualities must be rejected.[11] Boys may be starved for attention and put down as "sissies" if they cling and clamor for the closeness they need. Boys are traditionally taught to stuff all emotions through the often-heard retort, "Boys don't cry," or the more frightening threat, "I'll give you something to cry about." These early lessons teach them that it is not okay to show feelings, especially sadness or fear, so they stifle all emotion.

Most men are conditioned to not feel or express pain, grief, or hurt. The feelings of love, joy, and excitement also can get numbed. Anger, though, seems to be permitted and encouraged. Anger is cultivated through team sports where the goal is to "beat" the opponent as severely as possible. Boys learn that men are expendable, a commodity readily traded for "God and country." Many a five-year-old's life goal is to become a soldier, to fight.

As boys grow into teens they can easily become engulfed in a "culture of cruelty," in which they are victims, perpetrators, or witnesses of daily violence and humiliation.[12] Growing up in New York City, David was exposed to violence in the schoolyard, often between boys fighting with each other, and on occasion, was "mugged" on the playground by other boys, having to fight his way out by hitting one of the boys with a golf club.

Alan had similar experiences in England, where mobs of boys frequently clashed, violently attacking anyone they deemed unworthy, who supported a different team, spoke with a different accent, or had a different skin color.

Stephen's direct experience within the juvenile justice system brought him face-to-face daily with this "culture of cruelty" within peer and adult relationships.

Boys are socialized to fear each other. This is the truest definition of male homophobia: the fear of males, which is rampant in our relationships with each other—that to be too close to another boy may leave a boy labeled as "gay." In the maelstrom of puberty, such a label is social suicide. This creates a vacuum in which boys need emotional connection but may not have the social skills to obtain it in a healthy manner.[13] Parental guidance during this period is often fragmented at best. Fathers are often absent, either physically through divorce or work, or emotionally through their own shortcomings. Mothers can be extremely protective or overly dependent. Some boys feel emotionally abandoned at a very early age. Few boys survive childhood without some form of physical or emotional trauma, resulting either from the aggression of their peers or from the emotional separation from their parents.[14] Boys may learn to trust no one; instead, they "should" know how to take care of everything, how to fix everything.

It is not surprising, then, that so many men seek comfort with alcohol and other drugs, and that for many that initial comfort becomes a physical addiction. The void created by the trauma of boyhood can be filled, even if temporarily, by chemical enhancement. Pain can be numbed, shyness can be masked, and anxiety can be tempered. The need for connection without intimacy can be met. But what happens when the substances stop working, when the consequences of using them become unbearable? The unthinkable act of asking for help can only be overshadowed by the inability to receive it when it is offered.

Challenging Belief Systems: What Is It Like to Be Male?

This is the dilemma: how can we teach men, who are socialized to be incapable of sustaining trust, that their only hope of relief is to trust and to allow themselves to become vulnerable with their peers? Since this is counterintuitive, the transition can be difficult. In essence, when men begin their journey of recovery and change, they are asked to challenge the very core beliefs they have lived by. In our work we ask the question, "What is it like to be male?" The answers invariably include the following: lonely; isolated; armor-plated; judged; seen as a threat to women, children, and each other; aggressive; expected to perform, provide, and protect. When compared to what we ask of men in treatment (to be vulnerable, share emotions, take risks, cooperate, believe, accept others' ideas), it is easy to see how men could initially perceive treatment as threatening, if not impossible.

Thus, we believe that when providing care to men, the first goal should be to create an environment in which they can feel safe enough to allow themselves to open up to each other. In a safe space, emotional movement can occur. In a care environment, this may require having an all-male staff with which clients may interact, thereby breaking the cycle of relying on women to meet emotional needs.

There are five areas to address when helping men understand the "how and why" of their behavior. These areas, which will be explored in detail in some of the chapters that follow, are outlined here:

1. **Being a man**: We look at our societal standards of "real" masculinity. Dovetailing with the work of Paul Kivel[15], we examine the boxed-in stereotype that drives men's beliefs about themselves, the roles that men are expected to fill, and the anxiety attached to those roles. We talk about the limitations of forcing oneself to fit inside the box, and the incredible social price paid by those who dare to challenge the boundaries.

2. **Men and their family of origin**: We examine childhood messages and paint a picture of the dynamics that lead many men to a life of addiction and/or isolation. Where a man falls in

his family lineage, the role of fathers in men's lives, and how men can parent themselves if necessary are all addressed at length.

3. **Men and emotions**: The emotion most commonly identified by men is anger. Anger is generally accepted and often expected from men in our society, yet when inappropriately expressed it is destructive to the fabric of our culture. The distinction between the emotion of anger and the action of aggression, which is often blurred by early modeling, is an important one. Rage is often an expression of that anger. The yearning for power and control translates to anger in interpersonal relationships. Normalizing anger, untangling it from rage, recognizing its emotional cousins, fear and shame, and opening a dialogue helps to begin the process of learning to express anger in a healthy manner.

4. **Men and sexuality**: A quick scan of the newspaper tells us story after story of "men behaving badly" sexually, from movie stars to politicians and power brokers, engaged in rape, sexual assault, affairs, and other behaviors that range from the inappropriate to the criminal. Further, there is an underlying cultural belief that men should know about sex and that a "real man" can always please his partner. We discuss how exploring sexual values and mores in a safe setting can allow men to take an honest look at their beliefs. We address the issues of sexuality, sexual dysfunction, and sex addiction (or what we prefer to call "out-of-control" sexual behavior).

5. **The male spiritual journey**: We examine how to engage men in safe, nonthreatening, and nonjudgmental dialogue concerning spiritual matters. As men discover that spirituality is all about

connecting to life, the importance of spiritual development becomes more and more clear. Spiritual development requires that a man develop an ability to trust and eventually to rely on elements that are outside of himself. Most men, however, are taught from a very young age to be independent and self-sufficient. Although this is often an indirect correlation, men tend to conclude that to rely on anyone or anything else is a form of weakness that will shortly be exploited. Overcoming this dysfunctional early learning requires an environment where vulnerability and trust are redefined as *strengths* rather than *weaknesses*, and as acts of *courage* rather than of *cowardice*. As they spend time in this environment, men become more open to allowing themselves to clear the cobwebs from their spirits and begin to experience life and peace.

These components help form a framework for men to begin to identify with each other and help open the door to the possibility of community, which is often preconceived as unattainable or unnecessary. They also serve as the backbone for our work. We hope that this book will be useful as a therapeutic tool for the person in self-discovery and for the care provider.

Two: Growing Up Male

> "If you treat an individual as he is, he will stay as he is,
> but if you treat him as if he were what he ought to be
> and could be, he will become what he ought to be and
> could be."

—Goethe

H ow can men be emotionally oppressed in our culture? Men have economic power and are bigger than women and children, right? But how we perceive male hurt makes a profound contribution to men's compulsions and obsessions, whether drug abuse or addiction, out-of-control sexual behavior, and/or other behavioral problems. It affects men of all races and ethnicities. Teenage boys are dying from the male socialization process. There must be something systemic in our culture that pushes men into destructive behaviors. What factors in our socialization process create the discomfort in men that leads them to addiction?

When we're born, there's no evidence that there are inherent differences between men and women in our ability to feel, our ability to think and figure things out, our ability to connect and be intimate, and our ability to be close to other human beings. These abilities are universal and present at birth. We each have the ability to be spontaneous, the ability to love and to be loved, and we all have a strong yearning for power and control over our own destinies. In that respect, there is no difference between boy babies and girl babies. None of these abilities and desires has been shown to be gender-specific. Then something happens to us. Bit by bit, the male socialization process implants beliefs about maleness in us—shame-based beliefs that begin to chip away at our self-esteem, beliefs that chip away at our ability to be our natural selves.

What are these beliefs we're socialized to accept that tear us from our natural selves?

- Men aren't supposed to feel.
- "Good" men are strong, athletic, and physical.
- Men are expendable.
- Men aren't good at intimacy.
- Men and boys are basically violent.
- Men must be providers, protectors, and/or fixers.

These beliefs, born in our culture and transmitted through our media, literature, and the collusion of our society, tear us away from our true core selves. And there are powerful consequences of this training by our culture. These beliefs devalue men's lives.

Men are taught to believe that there are many things more important than themselves, like fighting for their country or protecting their families, or that they are only as valuable as they are good at providing for and protecting others.

Men are placed in competition with each other. They perceive situations as only win/lose, whether they are or not. Men constantly compare themselves to each other, as if all resources are limited and every situation is a zero-sum game, whether it is or not. This way of thinking turns all other men into potential enemies, not sources of support in our lives or, more importantly, life sources, such as our own male relatives.

And when men lose, they feel shame. These "particles" of shame collect like dust on the soul, dimming our zest for life. A man begins to separate himself internally between his inner "good guy" and his inner "bad guy." The culture rewards this competitive process through popular media and in life. The rewards are money and the resulting status.

Men are rewarded in this subtle and intense process of competition where nothing is more important than winning. But this kind of winning also implies losing. And men win and lose in two ways. We're rewarded if we win over somebody else, competitive sports being a primary example. But we lose out on noncompetitive activities for boys where everyone can win. This sticks out more sharply if you try to imagine what our culture would look like if we intentionally encouraged collaboration, respect, empathy, and teamwork as the priorities of a young man's life.

Men can permit themselves to entertain only the emotions that are consistent with the attitude to win, succeed, and achieve. How else can they accomplish those feats? Once a man begins to demand success and a "winner attitude," he must use aggression.

Our whole culture thrives on cultivating aggression in boys. Boys are exposed to cruelty among one another starting at age eight or nine, the same age that boys start paying more attention to their peers than their families. This boyhood aggression lasts until they reach about fifteen years of age. Until then, it's just "play," and "boys being boys." While they're still minors, it's as if our society gives young men permission to be aggressive. And what comes with this permission? First, poor impulse control in dealing with anger; second, depression from holding in anger in every situation in which they receive aggression or fear it.

These are the two main behaviors men develop to manage their emotions—aggression and depression. Fueling each other in a feedback loop, the vicious cycle of aggression and depression results in the cultural perception that men are insensitive, unemotional, violent, sex-driven, and basically inhumane.

These cultural messages were brought home to us when we were small boys, unable to protect ourselves. We grew up watching our fathers and mothers teach us about being men. And we saw and heard mixed messages: On the one hand, men should be strong and reliable. On the other hand, men are naturally insensitive, violent, and impulsive, and are not nurturing caregivers. At some point after we were born and declared boys, we started being touched in a nurturing way less and less, and in a "hard" way more and more, such as with a slap, pinch, or poke.

We were being toughened up.

This approach to gender creates a deep, unsatisfied hunger for attachment and affection, a pattern developed over the course of boys' formative years. Is it any surprise that many men develop a huge yearning to be touched? One of our culture's main sources of touch for men is sex, and it becomes the conduit through which they seek to respond to their yearning, often becoming compulsive about it. Data suggest that men are three times more likely than women to seek help for out-of-control sexual behavior.[16] A sexual compulsion rate of that magnitude occurring so disproportionately in one gender may reflect a social failure to meet boys' very basic need for attachment. We want to be touched; we yearn for emotional attachment. By the time boys become men, there may be a deficit that feels as if it can never be filled.

Let's return to the fact that there is no evidence for fundamental differences between men and women at birth—both need to love and be loved, to feel capable and powerful, and to be connected to others. The social script that casts men as too aggressive, too sexual, unable to show any emotion other than anger, and incapable of being caregivers to our children produces a constant stream of blows to our self-esteem. Instead of toughening us up, it leaves us vulnerable to anything that will ease the pain. It sets us up for addiction.

Why addiction? Because addictive behavior can numb our pain. If we do not transform this pain, we transmit it—onto ourselves and onto others. Men develop the disease of addiction at a rate three times higher than women.[17] After years of contradictory messages (don't feel, except anger, don't trust other boys, don't get too close to other boys), after years of not having had basic attachment needs met and being encouraged to buy into the attitude that girls are objects for pleasure and/or emotional nurturance, men live in contradiction with their true selves, in a world of hurt.

Most men have some level of underlying pain as a result of working so hard to do it right, to be perceived as a "good" man. And since we generally do not have internal resources to repair the hurt, we find something external, something "manly" and acceptable to repair or medicate our emotional pain.

Case Study: Ken

Ken is a fifty-four-year-old in a fifteen-year relationship with his partner. Over the last five years, Ken's partner has taken primary custody of her two grandchildren, an eight- and a nine-year-old. Child welfare officials have expressed concern that Ken's drinking is negatively affecting the children and have mandated Ken to addiction counseling if he wants to be involved in their lives.

Ken is a caring man who finds himself at a time in his life when he is ambivalent about having authorities inform, advise, help, or support him. Ken isn't one who can easily accept help or support because it stimulates feelings of shame that he cannot live as quietly and independently as he would like. He does not like being the focus of others' attention. His natural instinct is to fade back and avoid notice. That way he feels he can manage things his way, without others' advice or help. He becomes angry when he perceives people are telling him what to do.

Ken is fairly rigid about the "right" way to do things and will go pretty far, even to the point of conflict, to rationalize doing things his way. His history of accepting help has been spotty. He'll go to a few therapy sessions and then decide to go it alone.

Ken is intelligent, compassionate, and thoughtful, and has a nice way of thinking about other people. He has an interest in Buddhism, spirituality, and other healing entities. He struggles to know what to do about the needs of his adopted grandchildren. He is sensitive about being told the right thing to do for the children, especially because he believes that he is able to prescribe age-appropriate parental interventions for different situations. His strong concern for the kids has created a purpose in his life.

This purpose has given him the strength to step away from substances—to take the opportunity to stop using, even though he has found that very hard to do. Ken has stopped using all illicit drugs, such as marijuana and cocaine. He loves dancing, going out, being social; movement is especially important to him. He's ambivalent about quitting drinking because he doesn't believe that this particular behavior has had any effect on the children's development.

Ken's impulsiveness is triggered by his distaste for authority and for being controlled. This has caused him a great deal of anxiety, as well some medical problems he now struggles with. He is angered by any kind of authoritative intervention, which he sees as unwarranted interference. He feels hopeless about this attitude. Because Ken also doesn't trust peers, he is unwilling to participate in a group setting on a regular basis. This will make it extremely difficult for Ken to stay in recovery.

✏️ Exercise: Being a Man

Take your journal and a pen and put on some relaxing music. Find a comfortable seat in a quiet place where you will not be interrupted. Sit down and write each of the following prompts at the top of its own page. Then, under each prompt, identify and list some of the deep hurts you received in your past from the male socialization process.

1. What were some of your father's teachings or messages to you?

2. How did he teach you to "be a man"?

3. Are you ashamed of something you did to another boy when you were a teenager?

Now return to the page with your first prompt. Let yourself feel what was good and what hurt about that moment in your male socialization process. Think about how that moment connects to your present life and who you are now, and how it may have contributed to your addiction or compulsions. Repeat this process for the other two prompts.

Closure

I promise I will be proud to be a man who will seek the closeness in connection of every man, of every age, race, nation, and class. I will permit no slander or disrespect or blaming of any man for the hurts that have been placed upon him. I will seek to restore safety to all men to release the cruel hurts. I will fight to end and eliminate the burden of men's over-responsibility and overwhelming fatigue. I will cherish my birthright as a man, and I will cherish being a good, intelligent, courageous, powerful male human. I promise.

Three: Substances of Use

"To many, total abstinence is easier than perfect moderation."

—Saint Augustine of Hippo

Why do men find comfort in substances and destructive behavior? What is it that drives a man to seek out an altered state of mind? For many men there is a correlation between their initial introduction to alcohol or other drugs and their initiation into manhood. Drinking takes practice! It is not the taste of a substance that hooks, it is the effect. So what really happens when we seek an altered state of mind? There are many physiological changes that occur in the body when you add drugs, but what of the emotional and social effects?

Many men describe alcohol as a social lubricant. It may provide the initial freedom from the bondage of self-doubt and uncertainties:

uncertainty of how to act, how to fit in, how to "be a man." Time and again we hear men say that they "needed" a drink or two to quell the inner voices that prevented them from socializing. The problem for many men is that the line between "socially comfortable" and blackout is frequently, unintentionally crossed.

For many men, the use of substances is accepted as a rite of passage. Reports of college fraternity pledges dying of alcohol poisoning or drug overdose are all too frequent. Some of our most hallowed institutions of learning are more famous for their parties than for their faculties. For some men, these years of substance abuse are left behind upon graduation, and they adopt a life of moderate social drinking. For others, the substance abuse of their teens becomes the addiction that shapes their life's journey. Whether upper or downer, each drug has its own unique pathway to "somewhere else."

Somewhere else, anywhere else, is often preferable for a man who may be riddled with pain, shame, fear, and self-doubt. There may not be a definitive moment when a man moves from abuse to addiction. For some, a genetic predisposition has left them wide open to dependence. For others, years of abuse have left them physically unable to stop using. Either way, the outcome is similar: strained relationships, physical and emotional bankruptcy, missed opportunities.

Case Study: Chris

Chris had his first blackout at twelve years old. He had been sneaking drinks from his parents' liquor bar since he was five. He and his younger sister had long been in the habit of finishing up the many half-empty glasses on the mornings after their parents' numerous parties.

But this was different. He was at a party thrown by some older kids, and the alcohol was freely available. Chris had limited social skills. He was afraid of what others thought of him. To say that his family was dysfunctional would have been an understatement. His father was alcoholic, his mother a rageaholic.

The last thing he remembered about that evening was pouring a drink over one of his friends who was kissing a girl Chris liked but didn't know how to approach. Throw up. Fall down. Pass out.

This became a regular event for Chris. Drink. Throw up. Fall down. Pass out.

At school, violence was a daily occurrence. Being punched in the arm, thrown into a headlock, or kicked to the ground was routine. He was a less-than-average student, smaller than most of the other boys, and hyperaware that he didn't fit in. Gravitating toward the drinkers, the smokers, and the vandals, he began spending less and less time at home. He managed to avoid being arrested by sheer luck alone.

He became obsessed with pornography at thirteen years old and longed for a physical connection with a female. Having been frightened and confused by homosexual advances from older men, he had learned to be homophobic. He feared all men.

At fourteen he had intercourse for the first time. It was a horrible, humiliating, embarrassing experience for him. The alcohol he had consumed in order to raise his courage lowered his ability to perform. The fifteen-year-old girl, who was more experienced than Chris, grew impatient and verbally abusive toward him.

His alcohol consumption increased. The more he drank, the less he felt, and the more advances he made toward people who meant less and less to him.

He began smoking marijuana at fifteen. He also had his first real sexual relationship with a twenty-three-year-old neighbor. She would tap on his window when she was drunk and climb into his room. She taught him that sex could be pleasurable. She taught him about a woman's body. He felt good in her arms. Then she was gone. He wanted desperately to have a loving relationship. At fifteen years old he knew that he wanted to be loved, that he had never been loved. He had felt something like it in this woman's arms, and began to equate love with sex. He never considered that what had transpired was abuse.

At sixteen he again met a girl of his own age whom he really liked. When she became willing to be sexual he once again became impotent. She laughed. He cried with embarrassment and anger.

Chris vowed to never go through that again. He began to drink more frequently. He lost interest in pursuing sex and became voracious in his pursuit of getting wasted. His impotence lasted for a year. He could feel it whenever he became close to a woman he liked. After a year he discovered that he felt aroused around women he didn't particularly like. He discovered that he could be sexual as long as there was no emotional involvement—closeness without intimacy. His childhood had taught him that intimacy was dangerous, that it was painful. Now as he approached manhood he was incapable of intimacy. Now he sought physical gratification without risking intimacy.

He dropped out of school before his sixteenth birthday, left home, and lived for a short while with a variety of friends and relatives. He left each place after his drinking and drugging became intolerable to his host. Even the most loving friend or relative could only take so much. Chris threw up frequently and was sometimes incontinent while sleeping. He began to explore other drugs: methamphetamine, LSD, and cocaine.

He continued to smoke cigarettes and marijuana and drink alcohol on a daily basis.

Chris became dependent on women to rescue him. Never comfortable with more than superficial male relationships, he honed his skills to charm and conquer older women who could offer him food, shelter, and sex.

After his father died of addiction, Chris spun out of control. He was a social chameleon, adapting to the wants and needs of whomever he felt he needed for survival. One night in a bar he met the woman who was to become his first wife. She was fifteen years older, divorced, with four grown children, and was starved for attention. Chris performed his way into marriage. She took care of him, cleaned up after him, drove him home when he was too wasted to move, and didn't ask too many questions when he didn't come home. He treated her like a doormat. She loved him. Each was as debilitated as the other, and they needed each other. They spent six tumultuous years together, through countless affairs on his part. He continued to seek validation sexually every opportunity he had.

Finally he could pretend no longer. During a drunken blackout, he drove his car into a canal. It's tough to deny that there is a problem when your car is submerged and you are suddenly cold, wet, and afraid. He was arrested and charged.

Then came his first commitment to change, to stop drinking, to stop cheating, to change his life. He realized almost immediately that he couldn't stop. He called a twelve-step hotline and was told that the nearest meeting was in a church. He couldn't go to a church. He didn't believe in God. He hated religion. He began to think of suicide. It wasn't a new thought, just stronger than ever before. He wrote his wife a note, apologizing for how he had treated her, and headed to his favorite spot on the beach. On the way he picked up a bottle of vodka and refilled a prescription for Valium. On the beach he began drinking and popping the pills, slowly and deliberately. Eventually he passed out, not expecting ever to wake again. Five hours later, he woke up with the worst headache and the worst sunburn he had ever had. Even in suicide, he was a failure.

It was at that moment that Chris decided to seek professional help. He wound up in a drug and alcohol treatment center for twenty-eight days. The center was coed. Chris was assigned a female counselor and placed in group therapy with three women and five other men. He had a hard time staying focused, finding himself more interested in the females in the room, posturing and placating them, than in trying to share his feelings with the group. He wasn't even sure what he felt. The only feelings he was ever certain of were anger and fear. He was told he was in denial. He was told he was going to die unless he surrendered to his disease.

Each day clean helped him feel better physically. He was taken to twelve-step meetings but felt no connection. He told no one of his sexual escapades, of his countless affairs. He developed a crush on his therapist and worked hard to stay in her good graces. After he completed treatment he had a brief affair with a woman he met in the program. She got pregnant and wanted to start a life with him. He was still married and his life was becoming more unmanageable than it had been while he was using. The girlfriend moved away and later had a child he would never meet. His wife took him back . . . again.

For the next year he worked hard at staying abstinent and being faithful. But he had made no real connection to anyone in treatment, had not been able to stay focused enough to benefit from his sparse attendance at twelve-step meetings, and became sexually involved with the first "recovering" woman who showed him attention. Though he was not using, he was still behaving like the lonely teenager that he had been. When confronted by his now-desperate wife, he became angry and full of rage. After she filed for divorce, he felt as though he had nowhere left to go. So he went back to the one friend he knew he could count on—alcohol.

Despite asking for help, Chris had not been able to connect with the help offered. His drinking and drug use continued for two more years until he was hospitalized following an overdose of Valium. When it was suggested that he enter treatment again, he was reluctant. He felt it would be a waste of time and money. But the hospital social worker told him that she knew a place that was different, where he would really be able to find the help he wanted.

The second treatment center *was* different. Chris was in an all-male setting, with only male counselors. He was scared at first, as he had never been comfortable with other men, but he slowly came to see that he was not so different from his peers. He was challenged to take a good look at his life, at where he had been and where he was going. He was encouraged by his counselor to stay open to all possibilities. A spiritual counselor helped him work through his fear and anger toward God. The men played sports and games together. They laughed at and with each other and cried with each other. He began to experience a strange emotion—hope.

With the help of his peers Chris began to feel that it might be possible for him to recover. He completed treatment, continued in aftercare, remained connected to his peers, and stayed in recovery. He put aside his bias and attended twelve-step meetings and men's meetings.

He obtained a sponsor and began to work through the Twelve Steps. Different treatment, different results. What made the difference? What was it about the second treatment program that was successful? Was it simply that Chris was finally "ready to get well," that he had "hit his bottom," that he no longer was "in denial," was "resistant no more" (the excuses clinicians often give when a man drops out of treatment), or was there something about the quality of this program that worked?

As Chris's story unfolds, it seems apparent that the frequency, variety, and amounts of substances he used had a direct correlation to the frustration and emotional pain he experienced. Much of that frustration and pain is common to many men in our society. His story may be very different from your own, or from that of men you know, but each of us has a history that continues to unfold and affect our every interaction.

Knowing why a man became dependent is not as critical as his willingness to recover from that dependency, but it certainly can help to take a good look at the significant events over a man's lifespan and identify correlations in the types and amounts of substances he used and the consequences he incurred.

Exercise: Substance Use

In your journal, answer the following questions:

1. When was the first time you got drunk or loaded? How old were you and who were you with? What were the circumstances?

2. What feelings were affected by your substance use? How were you physically affected?

3. Write a timeline of any changes in your choices of substances. How old were you? What did you use or stop using? What was happening in your life?

4. How were your expectations of yourself affected by your use?

5. What are the major consequences of your use?

- Physical

- Emotional

- Spiritual

- In your relationships

- Financial

Four: Addiction: The Facts

"All philosophy lies in two words, sustain and abstain."

—Epictetus

Here are the facts about men and substance use and abuse:

- SAMHSA studies have found that the vast majority of American men over twelve years of age (82.6 percent) had used alcohol at least once in their lifetime. The data indicate that 9 percent of men reported heavy alcohol use (five or more drinks at one time in the previous month), compared to 2 percent of women. Approximately 34 percent of the sample reported using illicit drugs. Studies also indicate that drug use patterns vary significantly by racial and ethnic groupings.[18]

- Men are more than twice as likely to develop substance use disorders as women. Men begin using substances earlier than women[19] and have more opportunity to try drugs.[20] Men become intoxicated twice as often as women and are three to four times more likely to experience problem drinking and alcoholism.[21] These patterns cross all demographic lines of race, income, education, marital status, and geographic location.

- Men suffer far more adverse consequences of substance abuse than women.[22] Clearly, the social construction of masculinity plays a significant role in these statistics.

- Men's attitudes toward alcohol and other drugs tend to be generally less negative than women's attitudes. The use of substances is not viewed as a problem for men but rather as a rite of passage, a sign of true manliness. By contrast, substance use is more likely to be viewed as something for women to avoid due to increased sexual vulnerability. Moreover, such behavior is viewed as incompatible with female roles, including family and relationship expectations.[23]

- Co-occurring psychiatric disorders occur commonly among men. In one study, Swartz and Lurigo found that 55 percent of the men who were identified as having a substance abuse problem also experienced mental health problems.[24] Men often suffer from depression in conjunction with a substance abuse problem. On the other hand, men are not as likely as women to express their feelings of guilt, sadness, or worthlessness (all signs of depression) and may engage in reckless behavior as a way to deal with their depression. Men are also at greater risk of depression when they have experienced a trauma such as combat, an accident, or physical violence.

- Men are at greater risk for co-occurring medical problems, such as disorders of the liver, pancreas, and the neurological and gastrointestinal systems. Heavy alcohol use correlates with lower amounts of testosterone[25] and greater risk of prostate cancer.[26] Men who abuse alcohol are also more likely to engage in unprotected sex and are at greater risk of contracting HIV, hepatitis, and other STDs.

- Violence is closely associated with substance use and abuse among men; substance using and abusing men show high rates of violence.[27] The relationship between early childhood sexual trauma and substance abuse in men has been well-documented.[28]

- Men who use and abuse substances also tend to have higher rates of problems related to fatherhood and families. If divorced, they are twice as likely not to pay child support as those without substance abuse problems.[29] Substance abuse and violence may also be a factor in separating men from their families. The results of this alienation are dramatic: when men are not in relationships or do not have children they are less likely to complete treatment.[30]

Biological Aspects of Men and Alcohol and Other Drugs

Distinct differences in drinking and drug-taking behavior exist between men and women across cultures and ethnic groups, although the neurobiological action of psychoactive drugs is essentially the same for men and women.[31]

First, in terms of genetic factors and alcoholism, although men and women differ on many drinking-related dimensions, data are contradictory regarding gender and genetic risk for alcoholism. Jang,

Livesley, and Vernon reported significant genetic effects on alcohol and other drug problems only in men, whereas environmental factors have a greater effect on women.[32]

Contrasting findings are reported by Heath, who found no significant gender differences with respect to genetic contribution to alcoholism risk.[33] On the other hand, Walters suggests that the inheritability of a predisposition to alcoholism is stronger in males.[34] In Asian populations, Tu and Israel conclude that the female gender per se constitutes a major protective factor against alcohol consumption and alcohol abuse.[35] When taking all of the research into account, it appears that the risk of inheriting alcoholism is higher for men than women. On the other hand, environmental factors appear to be more strongly involved in alcoholism among women.[36]

Alcohol is known to affect the endocrine system, which does its work by means of various hormones that regulate bodily functions such as growth and reproduction. The part of the endocrine system concerned with male reproduction is called the hypothalamic-pituitary-gonadal (HPG) axis. The male reproductive system is governed by the interaction of the hypothalamus, a region of the brain, the pituitary gland, located at the base of the brain, and the gonads (testes). Alcohol, which affects all three parts of the HGP axis, is linked to low testosterone and altered levels of additional reproductive hormones.[37]

Additionally, as the HPG axis is affected, increased use of alcohol has a detrimental effect on the production of testosterone and is associated with increased levels of prolactin and estrogen in men. The impact of these changes is a condition called gynecomastia, which is the enlargement of breast tissue, atrophy of the testicles, loss of body and facial hair, and a general feminization of muscle tone. Other biological correlatives to substance abuse and dependence include:

- Changes to the immune system

- Chronic brain syndrome

- Wernicke-Korsakoff (W-K) Syndrome (understood to be caused mainly by the malnutrition often associated with alcoholism. People are at risk for W-K when they regularly drink instead of eating.)

- Korsakoff's psychosis (a particular manifestation or exacerbation of W-K Syndrome)

- Alcoholic pellagra, diabetes, gout, and respiratory disorders

- Gastrointestinal disorders, such as esophageal, stomach, and intestinal diseases

- Alcoholic pancreatitis, endocrine, and liver disorders

- Cardiovascular disorders and cancer

There is also a relationship between substance use in men and smoking and other disorders, such as sexually transmitted diseases, AIDS/HIV.[38] In addition to alcohol-related disorders, other drugs of abuse can result in significant biological concerns.

Although these effects are fairly consistent for both men and women, the fact that many men rarely see a physician or have routine medical checkups or care means that men entering an addiction treatment program may have several of these disorders, without ever having been screened for them. Hence, a thorough physical examination is an essential part of addiction treatment for men.

Five: Emotions

> "I was much further out than you thought. And not
> waving but drowning."

—Stevie Smith

Not Waving but Drowning *

For most men, freely expressing emotions was not encouraged as we grew up, with the exception of anger. We're out of touch with many other emotions: sadness, grief, loss, and even love. If you are a man, have you ever watched an emotional movie and surreptitiously wiped the tear in the corner of your eye away for fear of being seen as "emotional"? It is important for men to face a variety of feelings they may have been stuffing down through the years. This is best done "sideways," rather than directly. Instead of asking men to talk about their feelings, often it is more effective to address emotions through activities and rituals.

*By Stevie Smith, from *Collected Poems of Stevie Smith*, copyright © 1957 by Stevie Smith. Reprinted by permission of New Directions Publishing Corp.

When we think about our emotions, other than anger, we rarely express the full range of our feelings. Yet our emotions run the gamut from happiness and joy to depression and despair. It is important for men to explore questions such as:

- What makes you happy? What gives you a sense of energy, joy, peace?

- What brings you to life? What gives you meaning and passion?

- What emotions inside of you are waiting to come out? To be expressed?

- What emotions do you experience in your family, friendships, religious group, social life?

Facing our fears is also an essential step for men. As boys we are told to "suck it up, face your fears, never let them see you sweat," and how to distinguish between fears of real things and imagined fears. As men, we also need to face our real and imagined fears about life. "Will we have enough? What if I lose my job? How can I successfully support my family? What if something happens to one of the children?" Today, in a world filled with terrorist threats, random violence in our towns and cities, and natural disasters, men need to address questions such as:

- What do you fear about your job, your family, your lifestyle, your world? With whom can you share your fears?

- What skills do you have and use to deal with these fears?

- What are your views about health, about death?

- What does death mean to you?

- What emotions come to you when you have to face the mortality of family, friends, and even yourself?

- How do you live in the times when your life is changing?
- What emotions do you have when you do not know where you are or in what direction you're going?

Our definition of anger is that it is the voicing of our own reaction of displeasure or disagreement, in which we name the energy that exists within us and for which we take full responsibility. Rage, on the other hand, is the externalization of the same energy in blame, sarcasm, hurtful language, or physical assault with the goal of hurting or diminishing the blamed target. Anger is the one "legitimate" emotion men can express, although it is often inappropriately identified and expressed as rage. John Lee, in *The Missing Peace*, speaks to the manifestation of that rage and offers strategies for the appropriate expression of anger.[39] However, men and the people in their lives should not lose sight of what often lies beneath the anger: loss and sadness. Many men have a well of loss, grief, and sadness in their lives that they have never expressed. To get to these emotions, most men have to enter "sideways" through activities, rituals, films, and experiential therapies.

Exercise: The Grieving Cup

The Grieving Cup is a valuable ritual that is effective with men because it fulfills two purposes: it identifies something that is undeniable and true in men's lives, and it breaks through men's denial and reluctance to address emotions in a dramatic way. This activity can be done individually or in a group with a leader. Here it is written as a group exercise. At the end of the case study, we present it as if an individual were doing the ritual himself.

The group leader starts off with a small cup. It is best if the cup is made of clay and has an earthy feel to it, such as a Native American cup. Next, the leader introduces the ritual and gives those present the opportunity to participate or opt out, if they wish.

The group leader explains the ritual by saying something like, "Today, men, we will have an opportunity to remember an individual in our lives for whom we are grieving. I will pass this Native American pot around the circle, and you are to whisper the name of an individual for whom you are grieving. It might be the name of your deceased father, a friend that you've recently lost, a lost relationship, a loved one, or perhaps your addiction. When you breathe the name of that person into the pot, hold that person close to your heart and pass the pot to the next man in the circle. After all have breathed a name into the pot, I will take the pot back and bless it."

The following is a hypothetical interchange that might occur in a group. As the cup is passed around the circle of men, each member says to himself the name of an individual.

"My father, whom I have not seen in years."

"My wife, who recently died."

"My teenage son, whom I have not seen in a decade because of my addiction."

"My son, who died when he was ten years old."

"My best friend, who is ill with prostate cancer."

"My boss, who hates me because of my drinking on the job."

"My daughter, from whom I am estranged due to my addiction."

"My early years, which my addiction took from me."

"My son, who will not speak to me any more."

"Myself and all I wanted to be in life but which I failed to achieve."

The leader then holds the cup in two hands and raises it over his head. He says something like, "Having spoken the name of someone for whom you're grieving, I now dedicate these names. We hold them sacred. They have brought us great pain in our lives. We need to be released from that pain. We are now free from that grieving. Ashes to ashes, dust to dust. I now return these names back to the ground from which they came."

The leader then smashes the pot on the floor. Pottery shards splinter all over. The room is hushed. He says, "Men, we have returned these names to the earth. You are free. Who would like to express what is happening for him at this moment?"

The following is an exchange that might occur:

> **George:** "I feel a great sense of release, as if I don't have to hold on to that grief and pain any longer. After twenty years of being angry at my father for dying when I was ten years old, I can now let him go."

> **Michael:** "Wow, I did not expect you to do that. I am surprised, although I have a real sense of peace for the first time in my life. No longer do I need to hate my boss for what he did to me. It's gone."

> **John:** "I am really pissed off at you. How dare you! I breathed the name of my departed son into that pot. And you broke that pot. And then, to make matters worse, you stepped on the shards. That really makes me angry."

Dan: "When my father died, I was just a boy, a teenager. I never really got to know him. For all of my life I have held anger toward him for abandoning my sisters and me. Now, for the first time in my life I feel a sense of release. I can let him go."

Mark: "I am shocked at the way you threw the pot on the floor, in total disregard for my feelings. I guess anger is a common emotion for me, but that's not what I am feeling toward you (the leader) right now. I am feeling sad that this is what life comes to, a few spoken words, said in silence, and a broken life scattered on the floor. Is this what life is about?"

Craig: "I feel relief. My wife died recently, and I have held back the tears for too long. Is it okay to cry for her now?"

David: "Because of my addiction, my boss has come to resent me, my lousy lifestyle, my poor performance. I am at times a superstar at work, at times a terrible employee. I guess that's what I grieve the most. Although I breathed the name of my boss into the pot, I guess I really breathed the loss of myself, my potential, and my possibilities into the pot. I grieve for myself."

Lucas: "I have lived with so much pain in my life, physical pain from athletic injuries in high school and college. I used drugs and alcohol to relieve that pain. I never knew what they were doing to my body. I have never transformed my pain, only transmitted it onto others and my body. When you broke the pot, I felt pain relief—like that pain was being transformed for the first time in my life. Thank you."

Henry: "I am angry that you dashed so many feelings onto the floor. You seemed to have no respect for the value of the lives in the pot. Why did you do that?"

James: "Thanks for that sudden release. I needed something like that to break through my emotions, which I have kept bottled up in my own pot of self-pity. The pot is a beautiful image for me of my life, all self-contained, pretty on the outside, so many emotions on the inside; they remain there, inaudible, unobserved. When you broke the pot, you broke through that wall of containment."

Leader: "Let's talk about our anger. At what other things, people, or events are you angry? Who else in the group is angry now, at something or someone?"

John: "I am angry at you for dashing the pot. I guess I am also angry at the world. It just seems so unjust, so unfair. Why am I an addict? Why did my dad beat my mother? Why did he have to die at such a young age? I am angry at all of these things. I'm angry at my dad for dying, for abandoning me when I needed him, especially now that I am trying for the first time in my life to be clean and sober. He never really took good care of himself. He drank too much, too. He often beat my mother and me, but I still loved him. And just when I was trying to get my act together, he dies on me. That really pisses me off."

Leader: "John, how have you dealt with that anger and pain of loss?"

John: "I took my early anger and rage out on myself, through my drinking and drugging. But I don't want to do that anymore."

Leader: "If we don't transform our pain we transmit it. What would it mean to you, John, to transform your pain? Who else in the group has pain they'd like to transform?"

Lucas: "As I said earlier, I have a lot of pain I've never transformed. I take it out on my wife, the dog, my kids, myself. My addiction has numbed me to the pain. What does it mean to transform one's pain?"

Mark: "I need to transform my anger, too. I'm still feeling angry about what you did with the pot. How can I deal with that feeling? Tell me more about transforming pain. I don't know how to let go of the feelings I have for people who have let me down in life. It seems as if someone is always disappointing me."

Leader: "Tell us more about your disappointments in life."

In our hypothetical example, Mark might go into an extended statement about lost jobs, lost friends, lost loved ones, lost children, lost parents. The leader opens up the discussion to other group members to talk about disappointment and pain in their lives. The leader and the group discuss how they can transform their anger through letting go of their pain, surrendering to it, turning it over to their Higher Power.

The leader says, "Who else has these feelings? Who else has had pain in their lives? What have you done to transform your pain?"

Craig: "I have had so many physical ailments over the years. First my back went out, then I had high blood pressure, bad knees from sports injuries, and now I've been diagnosed with prostate cancer. It's like my body is falling apart. My alcohol and drug use made it easier to deal with my physical pain. I don't know what I am going to do without alcohol and painkillers. I want to transform my pain but I don't know how."

Matthew: "What has helped me is the First Step of my twelve-step fellowship, to be able to let go of my pain and to turn it over to my Higher Power. I saw I was powerless over my pain, that no matter what I did, I could not prevent problems from occurring. But I could at least not let it greatly affect me. That's how I've transformed my pain, and boy, have I had a lot of pain in my life."

Dan: "How do you let go when you've been so hurt? I need to learn because the problems I've had have just eaten away at me."

Leader: "Who can help Dan with his question? Perhaps we can go back to how we felt with the exercise earlier, recalling the feelings we had then."

Often at this point, group members discuss the pain they have felt in their lives. Many men speak of how they transmit their pain onto themselves through their substance abuse. This opens the group to a depth of emotions previously unattainable without some form of ritual that breaks through defenses and denial. The group discussion about this ritual goes on for several sessions as deep emotions are expressed.

At the end of the session, group members are invited to pick up a piece of shard and keep it as a token of the release of their pain. The leader asks the members to keep the shard and bring it back to the next group meeting to discuss what that shard has meant to them throughout the week.

This ritual illustrates the type of dramatic, authentic activities that can be used in groups with men. By this physical portrayal, emotions are quickly brought to the surface in a way that might not otherwise happen with men in therapy. Participants are given an opportunity to journal their reactions to the ritual.

As indicated previously, individuals can engage in a similar activity by themselves. Obviously, the emotions brought to the surface through the smashing of the pot may be intense, so it is best to have a friend or spiritual guide nearby to discuss these emotions.

The exercise can include the following questions to be completed in your journal:

1. What emotions are you holding that are eating away at you, that you need to release? For whom are you grieving?

2. Because what we fail to grieve becomes a grievance, to whom and in what way do you need to let go of long-held resentments, grief, feelings?

3. How long have you held these grievances? How have these emotions affected your life?

4. What do you need to do to let go of these feelings? What's standing in the way of your expressing these feelings?

✐ Exercise: Saying Goodbye

As an alternative to the Grieving Cup ritual, you might consider writing a goodbye letter to people in your life whose loss you still grieve. Begin by sitting quietly and relaxing your body, perhaps trying a form of meditation through breath and progressive body relaxation. The following is a form of relaxation exercise you might start off with.

Place your feet on the floor, put your hands wherever they are most comfortable, and close your eyes if you can. Take in a deep breath, as deep as you can . . . and exhale. Again breathe deeply, filling your lungs with cool air . . . and exhale, breathing out all that moist, stale air. Once more, inhale deeply . . . hold it . . . and exhale. Continue breathing deeply. Bring your focus to your feet, from the tips of your toes to your ankles, and as you focus on your feet, they become more relaxed. Now place your focus on your legs, from the ankles to the knees. As you focus on your legs from the ankles to the knees, they become more relaxed. Continue in the same manner up to the top of your head.

Continue with deep breathing, focusing on "peace" on the inhale and "surrender" on the exhale.

Now, to begin the process of saying goodbye to people in your life that you've been holding on to for far too long, visualize yourself standing in a thicket of woods. Look around. This may be a place that is familiar to you. Perhaps you were here as a child or as a younger adult. You can see the sun rays shine through the thick canopy of trees. You can feel the warm sunlight on your face. You can smell the earth, the decomposing vegetation. You can hear the buzzing of insects and whistling of birds in the trees. As you look around you notice that you are standing on a path that stretches out before you. You begin to walk along the path, and as you do you can hear the twigs and leaves crunching underfoot.

In the distance you can hear running water, and the ground begins to rise and then falls into a stream. You cross over the stream and up the bank on the other side. You continue on the path and the woods get thicker. Suddenly you see a clearing up ahead. It is a large clearing, about the size of a football field. In the middle of the clearing you can see a group of people standing in a circle, too far away to identify. As you get closer you begin to recognize some of the faces. These are the people who love or loved you, or who did not love you enough. Visualize who these people might be. Their faces are saddened, and there are tears in their eyes. What if they were gathered here because this was your funeral? What if you were never to see these people again in this life? What do you want to say to these people? What do you want them to know about your struggle, about your love for them, about your sorrow?

Write a letter to these people in your journal. Read to yourself what you have written to them. Is this enough?

✐ Exercise: Emotional Lineup

Answer the following questions to yourself, or write your answers in your journal:

1. What emotions do you most commonly feel, for example, anger, resentment, fear, anxiety, happiness? How have the emotions you feel changed in the course of your life?

2. For what or for whom do you need to grieve? Where do these feelings come from?

3. Write a timeline of events in your life that have brought you joy, happiness, peace, satisfaction, etc.

4. Write a timeline of events in your life that have brought you sadness, anxiety, depression, anger, etc.

5. Compare these two timelines in terms of their impact on your life and what you might want to do to focus more on the positive and less on the negative events in your life.

6. How have these events shaped your current emotional state?

7. What are the effects of these events on how you deal with your emotions now?

8. How have these events affected you physically, emotionally, socially, and spiritually?

Emotions—that's a tough one for us as men. As we have emphasized, often the only legitimate emotion men see expressed by their fathers or other men is anger, and that is most frequently released as rage. It is important for men to not use their anger to protect what is really lurking beneath the surface. Often, it is a feeling of deep sadness and loss, from sources long since buried in their lives. These exercises are simple ways to get in touch with the sea of emotions that rides below the surfaces of men's lives.

Men and Depression

Depression can strike anyone regardless of age, ethnicity, background, socioeconomic status, or gender. Research has shown, however, that depression is about twice as common in women than in men.[40] Researchers estimate that 12 percent of women (more than 12 million women) and 7 percent of men (more than 6 million men) in the US are affected by depression in any given one-year period.

For detailed information on the symptoms, types, etiology, and co-occurrence of depression and other illnesses, we refer you to *Men and Depression*, NIMH, NIH Publication # 03-4972.

Men experience depression differently from women and have different ways of coping with the symptoms. Men may be more willing to acknowledge fatigue, irritability, loss of interest in work or hobbies, and sleep disturbances than feelings of sadness, worthlessness, and excessive guilt.[41]

For many men, substance use and abuse and other addictive behaviors can mask depression, making it harder to recognize as a separate illness that needs treatment. Instead of acknowledging their feelings, asking for help, or seeking appropriate treatment, men may turn to substances when they are depressed, or they may become frustrated, discouraged, angry, irritable, and sometimes violently abusive. Some men deal with depression by throwing themselves compulsively into their work, attempting to hide their depression from themselves, family, and friends. Other men respond to depression by engaging in reckless behavior, taking risks, and putting themselves and others in harm's way.

According to SAMHSA, four times as many men as women die by suicide in the US, even though women make more suicide attempts.[42] In addition to the fact that the methods men use to attempt suicide are generally more lethal than those used by women, there may be other factors that protect women against death by suicide. Because men are less likely to seek treatment for their depression,[43] they are also more likely to die from suicide than to be diagnosed or treated for the depression that underlies the suicidal ideation.

Elderly men are particularly susceptible to depression and substance abuse. If men have been the primary wage earners for their families and have identified heavily with their jobs, they may feel stress and deep loss upon retirement—loss of an important role, loss of self-esteem—that can lead to depression. Men who have lost their jobs may also feel a deep sense of depression. Similarly, the loss of friends and family and the onset of their own and others' health problems as a result of aging can trigger depression in men. Healthcare professionals can miss depressive symptoms in older men, who may complain primarily of physical symptoms and are often reluctant to discuss their feelings of hopelessness, sadness, loss of interest in normally pleasurable activities, or extremely prolonged grief after a loss.

Thus, suicide is a special concern for aging men. There is a common perception that suicide rates are highest among the young. However, it is elderly men, particularly older white men, who have the highest suicide rates. The American Foundation for Suicide Prevention reports that the suicide rates for men rise with age, most significantly after age sixty-five, when the suicide rate for men is seven times that of women in that age group.[44]

About 60 percent of older suicide victims had visited their primary care physician within the month prior to their deaths, many with a depressive illness that has gone undetected.[45]

Only in the past two decades has depression in young men been taken seriously. Before puberty, boys and girls are equally likely to develop depressive disorders.[46] After age fourteen, however, females are twice as likely as males to suffer from depression or dysthymia. The risk of developing bipolar disorders remains approximately equal for males and females throughout adolescence and adulthood.[47]

Suicide rates for teenage boys are alarmingly high. In 2000, suicide was the third leading cause of death among young males, age ten to twenty-four. Among adolescents who develop major depressive disorders, an estimated 7 percent will die by suicide in their young adult years.[48]

The good news is that depression in men is treatable, with a good prognosis, through the proper use of medications, psychotherapies, electroconvulsive therapy, and/or herbal therapy. Family and friends can assist. Care providers need to be sensitive to the possibility of depression in men, especially in adolescents and older male adults. For more information, visit http://www.mentalhealth.samhsa.gov.

Section I Notes

1. Aaron Kipnis, *Angry Young Men: How Parents, Teachers, and Counselors Can Help "Bad Boys" Become Good Men* (Jossey-Bass, 1999), p. ix.

2. Ibid.

3. Ibid., p. x.

4. "Suicide Facts at a Glance," Centers for Disease Control and Prevention, 2010, http://www.cdc.gov/ViolencePrevention/pdf/Suicide_DataSheet-a.pdf.

5. Daniel Kindlon and Michael Thompson, *Raising Cain: Protecting the Emotional Lives of Boys* (New York: Ballantine Books, 1999), p. 170.

6. Stephen T. Russell and Kara Joyner, "Adolescent sexual orientation and suicide risk: Evidence from a national study," *American Journal of Public Health*, volume 91, number 8 (2001), pp. 1276–80.

7. "The 2008 Annual Homeless Assessment Report to Congress," US Department of Housing and Urban Development, 2009, http://www.hudhre.info/documents/4thHomelessAssessmentReport.pdf.

8. "Prisoners in 2008," US Department of Justice, 2010, http://bjs.ojp.usdoj.gov/content/pub/pdf/p08.pdf.

9. "Capital Punishment, 2010—Statistical Tables," US Department of Justice, 2010, http://bjs.ojp.usdoj.gov/content/pub/pdf/cp10st.pdf.

10. David M. Newman, *Sociology: Exploring the Architecture of Everyday Life* (Thousand Oaks: Sage Publications, Inc., 2008).

11. William Pollack, *Real Boys: Rescuing Our Sons from the Myths of Boyhood* (New York: Random House, 1999).

12. Kindlon and Thompson, *Raising Cain: Protecting the Emotional Lives of Boys*.

13. Pollack, *Real Boys: Rescuing Our Sons from the Myths of Boyhood*.

14. Ibid.

15. Paul Kivel, *Men's Work: How to Stop the Violence That Tears Our Lives Apart* (Center City: Hazelden, 1998).

16. Jennifer Schneider and Robert Weiss, *Cybersex Exposed: Simple Fantasy or Obsession?* (Center City: Hazelden, 2001), p. 83.

17. Russell Lemle and Marc E. Mishkind, "Alcohol and masculinity," *Journal of Substance Abuse Treatment*, volume 6, number 4 (1989): pp. 213–22.

18. "National Survey on Drug Use and Health," Substance Abuse and Mental Health Services Administration (SAMHSA) (2011), http://www.samhsa.gov/data.

19. Kathleen T. Brady and Carrie L. Randall, "Gender differences in substance use disorders," *Psychiatric Clinics of North America*, volume 22, number 2 (1999): pp. 241–52.

20. Michelle L. Van Etten and James C. Anthony, "Male-female differences in transitions from first drug opportunity to first use: Searching for subgroup variation by age, race, region, and urban status," *Journal of Women's Health & Gender-Based Medicine*, volume 10, number 8 (2001): pp. 797–804.

21. Lemle and Mishkind, "Alcohol and masculinity," pp. 213–22.

22. Richard W. Wilsnack et al., "Gender differences in alcohol consumption and adverse drinking consequences: Cross-cultural patterns," *Addiction*, volume 95, number 2 (2000): pp. 251–65.

23. Ibid.

24. James A. Swartz and Arthur J. Lurigio, "Psychiatric illness and comorbidity among adult male jail detainees in drug treatment," *Psychiatric Services*, volume 50, number 12 (1999): pp. 1628–30.

25. Mary Ann Emanuele and Nicholas Emanuele, "Alcohol and the male reproductive system," *Alcohol Research & Health*, volume 25, number 4 (2001): pp. 282–87.

26. Leslie K. Dennis and Richard B. Hayes, "Alcohol and prostate cancer," *Epidemiologic Reviews*, volume 23, number 1 (2001): pp. 110–14.

27. Jane Liebschutz et al., "The relationship between sexual and physical abuse and substance abuse consequences," *Journal of Substance Abuse Treatment*, volume 22, number 3 (2002): pp. 121–28.

28. Paige Crosby Ouimette et al., "Physical and sexual abuse among women and men with substance use disorders," *Alcoholism Treatment Quarterly*, volume 18, number 3 (2000): pp. 7–17.

29. Irwin Garfinkel et al., *Fathers Under Fire: The Revolution in Child Support Enforcement* (New York: Russell Sage Foundation, 1998).

30. Jonathan Rabinowitz and Sergio Marjefsky, "Alcohol & drug abuse: Predictors of being expelled from and dropping out of alcohol treatment," *Psychiatric Services*, volume 49, number 2 (1998): pp. 187–89.

31. Glen R. Hanson, "In drug abuse, gender matters," *Director's Column, NIDA Notes*, volume 17, number 2, National Institute on Drug Abuse, National Institutes of Health, US Department of Health and Human Services (2002).

32. Kerry L. Jang, et al., "Gender-specific etiological differences in alcohol and drug problems: A behavioral genetic analysis," *Addiction*, volume 92, number 10 (1997): pp. 1265–76.

33. Andrew C. Heath, "Genetic influences on alcoholism risk: A review of twin and adoption studies," *Alcohol Health and Research World*, volume 19, number 3 (1995): pp. 166–71.

34. Glenn D. Walters, "The heritability of alcohol abuse and dependence: A meta-analysis of behavior genetic research," *The American Journal of Drug and Alcohol Abuse*, volume 28, number 3 (2002): pp. 557–84.

35. Guang-Chou Tu and Yedy Israel, "Alcohol consumption by Orientals in North America is predicted largely by a single gene," *Behavior Genetics*, volume 25, number 1 (1995): p. 63.

36. Marc A. Shuckit, et al., "The clinical course of alcohol-related problems in alcohol dependent and nonalcohol dependent drinking women and men," *Journal of Studies on Alcohol*, volume 59, number 5 (1998): pp. 581–90.

37. Emanuele and Emanuele, "Alcohol and the male reproductive system," pp. 282–87.

38. National Institute on Alcohol Abuse and Alcoholism, "Alcohol and AIDS," *Alcohol Alert*, number 15 (2000), http://www.niaaa.nih.gov/publications/journals-and-reports/alcohol-alert.

39. John Lee, *The Missing Peace: Solving the Anger Problem for Alcoholics, Addicts, and Those Who Love Them* (Deerfield Beach: Health Communications, Inc. 2006).

40. "National Survey on Drug Use and Health," SAMHSA (2011).

41. Pollack, *Real Boys: Rescuing Our Sons from the Myths of Boyhood*.

42. "National Survey on Drug Use and Health," SAMHSA (2011).

43. Kivel, *Men's Work: How to Stop the Violence That Tears Our Lives Apart*

44. "Facts and Figures: National Statistics," American Foundation for Suicide Prevention, 2009, http://www.afsp.org/index.cfm?fuseaction=home.viewpage&page_id=050fea9f-b064-4092-b1135c3a70de1fda.

45. Ibid.

46. "National Survey on Drug Use and Health," SAMHSA (2011).

47. Carol M. Worthman, "Biocultural Interactions in Human Development." In *Juvenile Primates Life History, Development, and Behavior*, eds. Michael E. Pereira and Lynn A. Fairbanks (Oxford: Oxford University Press, 1993), pp. 339–58.

48. David Shaffer, et al., "Psychiatric diagnosis in child and adolescent suicide," *Archives of General Psychiatry*, volume 53, number 4 (1999): pp. 339–48.

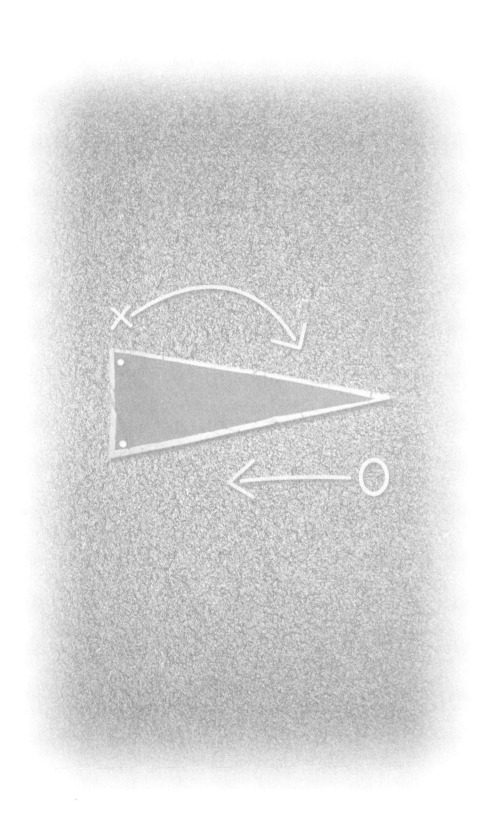

Section II: The Culture of Men

One: Men in Relationships

Men's Intimate Relationships

Acentral issue for all humans is finding ways of living with others, especially their partners, and redefining these relationships. Robert says, "I feel insignificant with my mate. There was a time in our relationship when roles were clearer. I worked on the family's financial needs; my partner took care of the house. Now, she is working, since I got laid off from my job. It's now so confusing."

Today, many shifts are taking place in role identities. This leads to role confusion for many men. This is especially so as men age. Men often find themselves interested in the more traditional female roles of nourishing and nurturing loved ones, while their partners may be task- and career-oriented. Let's not start applauding yet. Not everyone takes part in this role change, nor does everyone like it.

There are some questions men might ask themselves now about their roles and the important relationships in their lives:

- In what ways has your perception of traditional gender roles changed in recent years?

- How has your partner's role changed?

- What role changes might happen to you and your partner in the near future? Distant future?

Married men live longer, at least that's what the research says.[1] Men from the ages of forty-five to sixty-four who live with their partners are twice as likely as their uncoupled counterparts to live an additional ten years.[2] Being married remains the strongest association with male survival, even after accounting for differences in income, education, and risk factors like smoking, drinking, obesity, and inactivity.

Since men with solid relationships with women live longer, it is important to assess the quality of those relationships. The following are questions one could ask a man about his relationships:

- What are the primary relationships in your life?

- How would you describe these relationships?

- Do you have any close female companions with whom you share your inner secrets?

- What is lacking in your primary relationships? How could these relationships be different?

- What do you need to do to bring about these changes?

- Does your current relationship allow you to experience vulnerability, comfort, openness, and trust?

In developing new relationships with others, especially intimate ones, it is helpful to follow some tried-and-true steps to health:

- Become aware of the barriers that may exist for men between themselves and their intimate partners, especially barriers caused by sexism and homophobia, and work toward reducing or eliminating them. Reconciliation begins by seeking to understand how each partner feels in the relationship, what each wants and doesn't want.

- Be comfortable in relationships by putting aside anxiety about sexuality. It is a time to be honest with yourself and your partner about what you both truly want.

- Use affirmations such as, "I will start to participate fully in the emotional, physical, and relationship issues of my life, especially intimate ones, and stop asking my partner and friends to do more than their share." "I will develop one spiritual friendship with another person in the next year." "Today we begin anew. Today I will love you anew. Come with me on this journey. Grow old along with me."

Sex

Is there sex after recovery? There is a scene in the movie *28 Days* when a man in a group session asks the presenter when he can be sexual again. The presenter tells him to first get a plant, then a dog. If after the first year of recovery the plant is still alive, and after the second year the dog is still alive, then he can be sexual again. The man asking the question slumps in his seat, obviously feeling disappointed and confused.

Although this is a humorous movie scene, sexuality is a critical issue for most men, which in our experience is usually not addressed by care providers in men's recovery. Without addressing sexuality and intimacy as aspects of recovery, care providers may help to set the man up for relapse. In their youth, males probably sought to have a permanent erection from the age of eighteen to forty. But in their forties and fifties, sex can be troublesome for some men. Research shows that half of all American men experience impotence at least once after turning forty.[3] For men over forty there are significant changes in the occurrence of moderate impotence, meaning a problem with attaining and maintaining an erection about half the time they have a sexual encounter. Problems of declining sexual potency affect nineteen million men over forty in America.[4] Now, thanks to Viagra and Cialis, the frequency of impotence may be changing.

To explore the issue further, we invite you to ask yourself the following questions:

- What physical changes have you noted recently in your sexual life?

- To what extent are you concerned about changes in your sexual life?

- How frequently, if at all, have you experienced impotence?

- On a scale of one to ten, with ten being the best sex you have ever had and one being the worst, how would you rate your current sex life? How would your partner(s) rate it?

To have a more fulfilling sex life, there are changes you may want to try:

- Patience is pivotal. If you have the attitude of "penis-as-performer," you will inevitably fail. With patience, if you maximize the time you enjoy intimacy before you have an erection, your sexuality will contribute to your energy rather than deplete it.

- You no longer have to prove yourself as a young stud. It is time to graduate from Herculean sex to "surfing sex." It is like riding the crest of a wave, enjoying it in the ebb tide as well.

Men's Relationships with Men

Male friendships are also central in life. An inevitable sorrow of living longer is the diminishing circle of peers—colleagues and friends. Over time, we may lose friends through illness and death, but also through our own neglect of the relationship. As we lose friendships we lose a part of ourselves, the history, the legends we have shared, and the memories of who we once were.

Men who have identified the importance of having these relationships work to maintain them. As an example, it is helpful to look at the number of male friends you have today in comparison with the number you had twenty years ago. Many factors get in the way of maintaining friendships:

- Work responsibilities
- Family relationships
- Busy lives
- Lack of time and different priorities
- Fatigue
- Envy and competition

For some men, the competitiveness they might feel with other men may be a barrier to relationships and connection. One of the areas of greatest competitive vulnerability for men is money. Talking about one's income is the final taboo in western society. A man will never ask another man what he earns. Instead, we look at the symbols of income: cars, houses, perks, privileges, clothing, etc.—all external symbols of our "false self." Competition about money can be a great dividing line, limiting connection and vulnerability.

To be healthy, men need to outgrow this destructive competitiveness, whether centered on sports, salary, or penis size. It is important to "choose well one's friends, for in the end, we will become like them." If we have healthy, open relationships, we will become healthy and open. For most men, developing such relationships requires a new pattern of relating to others, a mutuality that demands equality. Friendship means letting down your defenses, showing that you are less than perfect, letting go of the need to be right, and trusting a friend with your heart. It entails a safe place to try out things, to stretch and grow, to be unashamed of what we say and think. Friendship demands candor, which is always speaking truth in love, based on a foundation of love and intimacy.

It is difficult for men to build this kind of relationship if they are competing with, ridiculing, and otherwise hurting other men. "Trash talking" between men may be a form of "wrestling" with one another, but it can be hurtful. Similarly, if you are afraid that your offer of friendship will be met with ridicule and hurt, you may be reluctant to embark on friendship with another man. It is important for men to make space and time in their lives for male friendships. To illustrate this point, David, one of the authors, noticed that recently he has been spending less time on the road, which had previously provided opportunities to see many of his male friends. Therefore, so that the friendships did not suffer from neglect, David suggested that ten of his male friends get together at a ranch in Arizona, à la *City Slickers*, and spend a week doing nothing except "being." This was a wonderful opportunity for these men, not all of whom knew each other, to renew and retain their existing friendships and to develop new ones. But it required David's commitment to get the group together and the members of the group's commitment to participate.

Being a better listener and spending time with other men helps men build communities in which they belong. Men can learn to be better listeners to their friends and be actively involved in identifying with, caring for, and thinking about men similar to and different than themselves. This involves understanding that other men have the same fears of emotional and spiritual intimacy, while also acknowledging that they all want the same thing: connection. This requires the willingness to make time in the midst of life for a male friend. An important side effect of this community with men is freedom from homophobia (fear of homosexuality that can take the form of being afraid of homosexuals, of being perceived as being homosexual, or of being homosexual), which can cause men to distance themselves from other men.

Research has shown that problems for men are often related to the strengths or weaknesses in their support systems. A primary task for men is to strengthen their support systems, that is, their relationships with the people in their lives (besides their partners) who will help them through whatever problems might arise. Men need to find different levels of friendships that can fill their life with significance, rather than relying on a particular person or group as the sole source of nourishment.

✐ Exercise: Looking at Your Support System

Here is a test of your support system.

Who is part of your support system (family, friends, extended friendships, work colleagues)? Using a scale of one to five, (one means strongly disagree, two means disagree, three means neither agree nor disagree, four means agree, and five means strongly agree), give a rating to the following statements:

- I can usually contact a friend when I need support.

- My friends check in on me periodically, especially when they know I am going through a tough time.

- My friends remember the details of what I am going through.

- I feel comfortable and safe when I am with my friends.

- These friends respect my needs and requests.

- My friends and I have similar outlooks on life.

- My friends and I take turns sharing equal time to talk. Our conversations are rarely one-sided, focusing more on one or the other, unless one of us needs help.

- My friends allow me time to talk about the issues I am working though.

- I feel energized when I am with my friends.

- I feel heard when I share my thoughts with my friends.

- I can discuss difficult topics and personal issues with my friends.

- My friends are honest with me when giving feedback.

- My friends give advice only when I ask for it. They support my decisions and help me take the actions I need to take.

- I feel comfortable expressing all my emotions around my friends, such as anger, fear, sadness, hope, joy, and excitement.

- My friends understand what I am going through.

- My friends allow me to be where I am on my journey.

- My friends give me insight that helps me see things from new perspectives.

- My friends and I celebrate good times together.

- I feel I have a good, solid, reliable support system.

Total points:

If you have between seventy-five and ninety-five points, you likely feel well-supported by family and friends. If you scored between fifty-one and seventy-four points, you feel some support from friends and family. If you scored between forty and fifty points, your support system may be of moderate help to you, but you may need others in your life. If you scored below forty points, your interactions with your family and friends may be doing more harm than good. Take a good look at why you are relying on these people for support. Maybe you need to seek out others for help.

How does one build a stronger support system, especially with the time pressures under which men operate? It requires a degree of intentionality. This may not mean gathering at a ranch in Arizona, but may require similar attention to getting together: face-to-face, email, telephone, Skype, etc. Here are some ideas to strengthen these bonds:

- Reach out to those you wish to bring into your support-system circle.

- Meet for breakfast, go for a walk, invite a friend to go with you to a meeting (twelve-step, faith, community, civic gathering, etc.).

- Join a support group of like-minded individuals.

- Seek professional help to determine what the barriers are that may be keeping you from finding friends and family.

- Seek people with whom you can share hobbies, special interests, crafts, art, exercise, music, games, or spiritual direction.

- Offer help at a social service center in your town.

- Go where healthy people go.

It helps to nurture your friendships by engaging in conversations of ideas, insights, questions, and/or fears that may be floating around in your head. Requesting input from others and exploring their thoughts and reflections is a good start.

If you find yourself at the other end of the conversation, it is important to practice presence and simple listening, without judgments, assumptions, or the need to fix others' problems, and without belittling or dismissing their feelings. You can support your friends in their journey and their proposed plan of action, celebrating the journey with them and enjoying their success by staying in the present moment.

In sum, there is a cost to maintaining love and relationships, and it may require a change in attitude. The payoff is finding new ways of loving and being loved. To gain this reward, a man needs to create a world in which he can laugh, love, work, and play without fear of judgment; a world of celebration, not accusation, apology, and unexamined assumptions. The people we love are not only in our memories, they are in our presence.

Two: Family of Origin

"Could I climb the highest place in Athens, I would lift my voice and proclaim, 'Fellow citizens, why do you turn and scrape every stone to gather wealth and take so little care of your children to whom one day you must relinquish it all?'"

—Socrates

A man's experience as a child can color his whole life. The role models who set the stage endow the child with a heavy, yet often invisible, responsibility. How a father treats a mother, how he treats his children, his work ethic, his religious beliefs, his eating habits, his drinking/using habits (or other manifestations of addiction), his political beliefs, his bigotry or egalitarianism—these all can have a direct impact on his offspring.

Many factors affect a boy's upbringing. For approximately half of the men born in the past thirty years, divorce colors their early home life. Given that often children in divorce are placed in the care of their mothers, many men were raised primarily by their mothers, with weekend or absent dads. Remarriage, stepparents, and stepsiblings often create confusion, emotional withdrawal, and a general lack of stability. For a boy to carve a sense of what it is to be a man from such a splintered family tree is a difficult task indeed.

Some are fortunate enough to have male role models from outside of their nuclear family who help them with their transformation. Others struggle through adolescence, reaching adulthood with no blueprint of what being a healthy man looks and feels like.

Even when Mom and Dad stay together, often there is little connection with Dad, who is either absent through work or emotionally absent through his own lack of a healthy parental role model. Many men, therefore, are essentially raised by their mothers. Mom is looked upon to meet all emotional needs.

At the Men's Gathering workshop in Mentone, Alabama in 2005, John Lee and Robert Bly both spoke of the need to heal the relationship with mother. They posed the question: "Whose son are you? Your mother's? Your father's?"

They hypothesized that if the childhood relationship with and emotional dependence on the mother are not consciously released, then a man can have no successful primary love relationship. There is no emotional room for healthy love if a man's head is still focused on pleasing Mom. This is manifest in the epidemic of men who are unable to engage in a healthy intimate relationship. The sky is full of aging Peter Pans, circling bewildered and embittered women who are left wondering where all the "good" men went.

John Lee has an exercise designed to help men release the baggage of their relationships with their mothers (PEER Training, Inc.). In this exercise he has a man sit facing him, holding his hands. He then encourages the man to close his eyes and say the following:

"Mom, I need to let you go."

"Why do you need to let me go?"

"I need to let you go because . . ."

"What else?"

The pattern is repeated until the exhausted, emotionally spent man has nothing left to release, and ends with him saying, "Goodbye, Mom."

If Mom or Dad had a problem with alcohol or other drugs, or if the family home was chaotic, certain roles may have been assumed by each family member. These roles were captured by Sharon Wegscheider-Cruse, who skillfully detailed how they help family members both to grow up successfully and to appear as healthy as anyone else.[5] Each role has its purpose, its strengths, and its needs for transformation. The roles are:

Family Hero: He is the one who can see and hear more of what is really happening in the family and begins to feel responsible for the family pain. The role of Hero is to provide a sense of "self-worth" for the family. Family Hero needs to learn to ask for and take what he needs, to learn to accept failure, to relax, and to focus on self and stop "fixing" family.

Scapegoat: He is the one who is in the public eye. Having learned that he must perform, he gets much of his needed attention in destructive ways. The role of the Scapegoat is to provide a distraction from the family. Scapegoat needs to get through the anger to the hurt and to learn to negotiate instead of rebel. Scapegoat strengths: realistic, insightful, sensitive, and courageous.

Lost Child: He is the quiet one who never causes trouble. He feels hopeless and unimportant. He is often confused and fearful. He has learned to not make connections within the family. The role of the Lost Child is to offer relief. This is the one child the family doesn't worry about. Lost Child needs to reach out, deal with loneliness, face pain, and make new close relationships. Lost Child strengths: patient, creative, and independent.

Mascot: He is tense, anxious, and often overreactive. He defuses explosive situations by focusing attention on himself. He becomes a silly adult, whose relationships are often shallow and flighty. The role of the Mascot is to provide fun and humor. Mascot needs to take responsibility, to risk being serious, and to be assertive.

Because of the self-delusion and the compulsive nature of these behavior patterns, family members take them into every other relationship. Nonetheless, roles that were rigidly held in childhood can be changed in later years, depending on the needs of a given situation.

Exercise: Family Roles

Do you recognize yourself in any of the roles listed above? Answer the following questions:

1. What was your role in your family?

2. How has the role you played as a child affected you as an adult?

3. How are these roles being played out with your own children?

Lucia Capacchione, in *Recovery of Your Inner Child*, hypothesizes that in each of us lies a vulnerable child.[6] Her work promotes reconnection with that child by providing a blueprint for examining childhood wounds.

Her use of nondominant handwriting and drawing, although not advised without clinical supervision, has a therapeutic effect of breaking through the intellectual wall we often build to protect that inner child.

✏️ Exercise: The Family Genogram

A genogram is like a family GPS. Take a blank sheet of paper and map out your family. Use circles to denote the females and squares to denote the males. Draw lines between each to represent the nature of the relationship. If the relationship is positive, use a solid line. If it is negative, use a broken or dashed line. Create as large a genogram as you wish, branching out into uncles, aunts, and cousins if you have them. The object is for you to gain a realistic perspective of your family relationships and how your own relationship patterns were developed.

Answer the following questions:

1. Who were you closest to in your family?

2. Who did you fear the most?

3. What did you learn about relationships from your family?

4. With whom do you share behavioral traits?

✏️ Exercise: The Family Home

Turn to a blank page in your journal and draw a picture of the house in which you grew up. There may have been several houses, but draw the first one that comes to your mind. You may draw a floor plan if it works better for you, but the idea is to jog your memory and return to that place. What happened in that house? Draw yourself and your family members: Mom, Dad, brothers, sisters. Put yourself in any room or any part of the yard that holds energy for you. As you sense yourself there, answer the following questions:

1. Why did you place yourself where you did?

2. What happened in this place? Was it painful or was it joyful?

3. How did whatever happened here affect your life?

4. Who protected you at that time?

5. Who protects you now?

Patterns of behavior that served to protect us as children often present as liabilities in our adult lives. The same coping mechanisms that kept us from the wrath of those older than us who were tasked with caring for us but who may have perpetrated harm on us can keep us from developing healthy primary relationships. Perhaps you learned as a child that it was dangerous to tell the truth. Maybe there were times when telling the truth led to physical or emotional abuse. The boy who gets spanked for spilling his milk will soon learn to say anything to avoid that spanking: "The dog did it" or "My baby sister did it"—deflect, obfuscate, deny.

Case Study: The Liar's Path

Tom told lies. He lied when it would have been just as easy to tell the truth. Lying was a survival skill for Tom. When he was a boy he had been punished for telling the truth. Once. He never forgot it.

There were occasions as a child when he would brag about his family, making up grand stories of exotic vacations, swimming pools, and boats. Other times he would pretend that he had no family, telling people that he was an orphan or an only child. As an adult, he exaggerated his abilities and skills in the work environment, often finding himself faced with the truth only after he had created a mess.

It was in primary relationships that Tom's lying became most pervasive. Sometimes overt, often covert, but always present. He had, from an early age, been taught that if he was to be happy, then he had better find someone to take care of him. He also learned from his father that it was okay and even expected that a man would cheat on his wife. This set the stage for a life of doomed relationships, always ending in bitterness and tears. Tom, always seeking a "woman to take care of him," would frequently overlap his affairs, beginning a new one before ending the last. He blew through two marriages and countless shorter-term relationships because of his reckless attitude toward commitment.

When he finally found his "dream mate," Tom also found that the patterns of a lifetime were not necessarily put aside at will. Despite his best intentions, and often, seemingly against his own will, he continued to lie. Even when there was no possible gain from not telling the truth, he would lie. He often believed his own stories to the point of not knowing his own reality. Countless attempts to be "completely honest" with his mate led to frustration. It seemed that there was no solution. He felt as though he kept repeating the same mistake; only the details changed. It took several years of effort, counseling, and a patient, tenacious partner to finally begin to break the pattern.

Exercise: Honest Living

In your journal answer the following:

1. Where have you been dishonest in your life, if anywhere?

2. How has your dishonesty served you? How has your honesty served you?

3. How has your dishonesty harmed your relationships?

Practice honesty as you move through the day. Where does this seem more difficult? What feelings surface if and when dishonesty enters your relationships?

Three: Sexuality

"The fountains mingle with the river
And the rivers with the Ocean,
The winds of Heaven mix forever
With a sweet emotion;
Nothing in the world is single;
All things by a law divine
In one spirit meet and mingle.
Why not I with thine?"
Love's Philosophy

—Percy Bysshe Shelley

An open discussion of sexuality is not on the top of most men's "to-do" list. It is a rare man who will openly discuss his fears and uncertainties about his sex life. Looking at sexual values and mores in a group setting often removes the bravado factor and allows men to take an honest look at their beliefs. Issues of sexuality, sexual dysfunction, and sex addiction, although often taboo subjects, are of primary importance to any man struggling to sort out the truth from the messy messages of their youth.

For both gay and heterosexual men, their earliest sexual experiences were fraught with performance anxiety and were far from the Olympian pinnacles of pleasure that they had expected. Peer pressure, the mandate to succeed, the expectation that they should know what to do, and the fear of failure do not make for a relaxed and focused union. For others, the pressure to lose their virginity might have been overwhelming. Poor choices in partners, lack of awareness or experience in the use of birth control, and the ever-present fear of rejection have always been recipes for sexual disaster.

Sex sells. Madison Avenue executives know this. Fortunes are made in advertising aimed at man's inherent appetite for sex. Weight loss, exercise, and hair-loss prevention products have grown into giant industries with the primary aim of helping today's man stay sexually viable. In the past two or three years it has become impossible to escape the myriad clever commercials for medications that promise to eradicate "erectile dysfunction." It was an astute advertising executive who thought of saying, "Be sure to call your doctor if you experience an erection lasting more than four hours." Suddenly it's cool to have "ED," which reportedly affects 20 million men in the US alone. Most of the advertising promotes only one aspect of a sexual relationship—the physical component. But what of the emotional, societal, or spiritual components?

One of the fastest growing industries in the world is Internet pornography. More than 60 percent of all visits and commerce on the Internet involve a sexual purpose.[7] Voyeurism on an international stage, increasingly with "real-time" video and audio components, promotes sex without intimacy. Physical gratification for some becomes full-blown addiction for others. What may begin as a seemingly harmless curiosity—the slippery slope of Internet pornography—can result in destroyed relationships, unfulfilling sex lives, complete emotional, social, and financial wreckage, as well as loss of any reality base.

The following exercise is designed to help you examine your sexual beliefs, history, and fears.

Exercise: Your Sexual History

Answer the following questions in your journal:

1. How was the subject of sex addressed in your family?
2. Who taught you about sex?
3. How old were you when you had your first sexual experience?
4. How many sexual partners have you had?
5. Did you ever coerce or force anyone to have sex with you?
6. Have you ever been forced or coerced into having sex with someone else?

Sexuality and Manhood

Joe is completing his twenty-eight-day stay in a treatment program after detoxification. He's been in recovery for four weeks. His wife, Mary, is looking forward to Joe's coming home clean and sober for the first time in years. During family week at the treatment center, Mary asked about how recovery might change their marital relationship, what impact it might have on parenting issues, and how they could begin to develop greater intimacy and sexuality. Robert, the counselor, in all seriousness, told Mary and Joe to "keep your legs crossed for a period of time—we recommend a year—so that good, long-term recovery can be established." Mary turns to Joe and thinks, "Yeah, right! For the first time in ten years he'll be clean and sober and we can have healthy sex again. And this jerk is telling us to keep our legs crossed? No way!" Joe is thinking, "It's show time. Now that I'm in recovery it's time for Mary and me to play sexually."

The way Robert and the staff of his program treat sexuality is typical of many treatment centers, which send either an incorrect or misleading message about sexuality, intimacy, and recovery. For many addicts, sexuality has at best been buried under layers of pain and abuse. Telling them to "keep it buried" does not work. It is likely that many counselors approach sexuality in this way because they have had little or no training in sexuality. Sexologists and sex therapists have excellent training in how to deal with sexuality. Unfortunately, most of them admittedly know little about substance abuse. On the other hand, addiction counselors have excellent training and experience in dealing with substance abuse, but little training in sex counseling. So substance abuse counselors either rarely bring up the subject of sexuality in sessions, especially in early recovery, or, as in the case of Robert, they provide well-intentioned, but misinformed, information and recommendations.

The interrelationship of alcohol use and sexual activity has been established for millennia. Moreover, there is widespread awareness that alcohol abuse can cause or exacerbate sexual problems. In fact, the rule should be that if you see one, look for the other. If a man is alcoholic, he will likely experience some sexual difficulties as well.

Sexual problems in substance abusers are multifaceted, affecting all aspects of functioning. Because sexual problems may have an organic etiology, primary care medicine, as well as specialties such as urology, gynecology, and neurology, need to be involved in screening, assessment, diagnosis, and treatment. The high incidence of physical trauma, such as rape or incest, among substance abusers means that legal professionals are often included in the treatment process. Addicts' sexual problems have psychological and relational effects that may require social work, psychiatry, clinical psychology, and all forms of counseling (the "talk-therapies") intervention. It is truly a problem with a multidimensional and interdisciplinary focus.

Substance-abuse counseling, with its dual interest in achieving abstinence and in the client's general emotional and relationship health, can and should play a significant role in responding to the sexual problems of clients. Addiction professionals are in a unique position to ensure that other disciplines are sensitive to the particular needs of the client and that services addressing sexual issues are provided in a manner that confronts the primary problem of addiction and enhances the client's potential for recovery from addiction.

Addiction professionals can also be advocates for the creation of specific intervention programs for the addict, his sexual partner, and other individuals such as family members and victims of sexual assault occurring under the influence of substances. The role addiction professionals can play in dealing with sexual problems of their clients is limited only by their lack of knowledge, experience, and clinical skills.

The following is a summary of sexual dysfunctions related to the use of particular drugs by men and women:

Alcohol can cause significant reduction in latency of penile tumescence (slower erections), decreased number and rigidity of erections, and high rates of semi-erections. While alcohol reduces inhibition, which can increase desire, it can also obstruct testosterone production, which in men reduces sexual desire. This happens in a serial fashion, with increased desire in the early stages of inebriation, declining into decreased desire and physical sexual suppression. This is discussed more fully below:

- Sedatives and hypnotics can cause depressed libido over time; consumption can result in absent libido, decreased testosterone levels for men, and, concomitantly, impotence as well as increased prolactin levels. When prolactin increases, it may result in a feminizing process (e.g., breast enlargement, change in muscle tone and body hair.)

- Cocaine has a biphasic effect; the person may initially feel sexually euphoric, but over time there is decreased libido, inhibited sexual desire, and impotence.

- Amphetamines can cause anorgasmia, with similar effects as with cocaine.

- Marijuana use can decrease testosterone levels, contribute to gynecomastia, increase prolactin levels for men, and possibly promote fetal abnormalities.

The consumption of alcohol and/or other drugs has an inverse relationship to sexual performance for men. The more a man consumes, the lower his ability to have an erection and orgasm. This phenomenon is not influenced by expectations, for although sexual desire for men is greatly affected by the setting and circumstances of alcohol consumption, the ability to perform does not improve with increased drinking.

Thus, increased alcohol and drug use leads to decreased libido and disinterest in one's sexual partner.

In addition, both alcohol and marijuana can cause feminization in men. This is a result of gynecomastia and testicular atrophy due to either a disturbance of the hypothalamic-pituitary axis or peripheral changes in the man's liver functioning. The symptoms of gynecomastia are enlargement of the breasts, decrease in muscle tone and body hair, and a feminization of the pubic hair area. The net result is changes in the gonadatropins. These changes in turn increase responsiveness to estrogen in men and decrease testosterone levels, as well as penile tumescence and diameter, which then become insufficient for penetration during intercourse.

Impotence is not uncommon for men, nor is it unique to men who abuse alcohol and/or other drugs. All one needs do is turn on the television almost any time of the day and watch commercials for erectile dysfunction (ED), the new euphemistic way of speaking about "impotence." Thirty million men have experienced partial or temporary ED. By the time the average man reaches forty years of age, he likely has experienced at least one episode of ED in his lifetime. ED is most often a result of overconsumption of alcohol or other drugs, fatigue, stress, relationship conflict, depression, or any number of emotional and psychological factors. As men age, ED rates rise. By the age of sixty-five and over, 25 percent of men have sought help for impotence. Organic factors contribute to impotence in men as they age: vascular disease, diabetes, hypertension, kidney disease, MS, heavy smoking, pelvic trauma, spinal cord injury, and hormonal abnormalities. Many of these factors are interrelated and can also cause problems elsewhere in men's lives.

Finally, there is a high correlation between the use of certain medications and impotence. These medications include antihypertensives, beta-blockers, psychiatric medications such as antidepressants and benzodiazepines, Phenobarbital, and Dilantin. All of these factors must be explored before a complete and reliable diagnosis of erectile dysfunction can be made.

As impressive as the statistics are, ED may be underreported. It has been said that if you really want to know whether a man is experiencing impotence, ask his partner, not him. It is difficult for a man to say, "I am having trouble getting it up." Such a statement may be a blow to his ego. The man who abuses substances may be too intoxicated even to know if he is having trouble with impotence.

Exercise: Substance Use and Your Sex Life

Answer the following questions in your journal:

1. In what ways has your substance use affected your sex life?

2. How has a diminished or diminishing libido affected your self-esteem?

3. How has a diminished or diminishing libido affected your relationship with your significant other?

4. In what ways, if any, might you benefit from a diminished libido?

Four: The Male Spiritual Journey

"I live my life in growing orbits,
Which move out over the things of the world.
Perhaps I can never achieve the last,
But that will be my attempt.
I am circling around God, around the ancient tower,
And I have been circling for a thousand years,
And I still don't know if I am a falcon, or a storm, or
a great song."

—Rainer Maria Rilke

"Before enlightenment, chop wood, carry water.
After enlightenment, chop wood, carry water."

—Zen Proverb

The spiritual journey of the male includes two major spiritual tasks: discovering what he is to be and moving into a deeper inner life, with a sense of self and the world. The two essential questions in life for men are *how to live* and *why*. It is as simple (and complex) as that. The temptation is to wallpaper the empty spaces of our lives with work, not providing the necessary balance among service, work, and avocation. But the true male spiritual journey is to grow in grace, not just in doing more things.

Male spirituality involves not just one compartment of life, but the deepest dimension of the person a man is made to be—his ultimate questions, hopes, fears, and loves. It gives him meaning in living by addressing life's questions of self-worth and significance. It reveals the mysteries of living, the realization that life's ultimate meaning cannot lie in speed, youth, consumerism, achievement, and physical beauty as defined by our culture.

This chapter explores the male spiritual journey. It first explores the downward, or inward, journey calling men to face their limits and wounds, the essential journey of letting go of control. The journey takes them into their desert spaces, the alone times where they confront who they are, their true selves. The chapter then turns to the interplay between the outward and inward components of the journey, to finding new sources of joy and refreshment in life. This involves a man getting in touch with something greater than himself.

Be careful of the man who tells you life is one joy after another with no desert times. He is fooling himself. Digging deeper requires time alone in the desert of his spirit and periods of feeling lost. Men don't like to be lost; after all, men are problem solvers who never ask for directions.

Male spirituality involves time in the desert, the darkness, the wilderness, from which he is reborn into something new and wonderful.

Men recoil from the idea of going downward and inward, for they fear descent and decline. They fear they will be insignificant when they leave behind the power, possessions, and prestige that drive them.

In the first part of a man's journey he finds himself filled with ascent, being in control of the outward parts of his life. In the second half of life a man goes inward, giving up his efforts to control, digging deeper to new sources of refreshment. To get there, he must go through his brokenness and woundedness.

Male spirituality is primarily a journey of acceptance of his own limits, realizing that no one can have it all; of seeing the limits of his power and exploring the language and contours of his pain. The journey takes men through the dark night of the soul of pain to the light of trust. All men experience some pain through wounds in relationships, career setbacks, physical illness, and deaths of friends and colleagues. What they do with that pain determines how they will live.

The desert is not just a place, but also a state of being. Most of a man's daily life is filled with blasts of the boring and ordinary. Yet, in the deserted, abandoned part of his day, when he feels most alone, a man faces the ultimate question of life, "Why am I here?" It is in the desert that men can begin to answer that question.

Further, the dark night of the soul is not always a dread-filled and depressing experience. The real meaning of the term "dark night of the soul" is that things may be obscure. We cannot see or grasp what is happening. It is a sense of unknowing, of mystery. In those dark times we need to trust someone else to be our guide.

Spirituality based on brokenness demands rethinking what it means to be a man. A man is not solely his faults, his body's diseases, or his role (being a father, husband, son, or employee). The fact is that each man is much more than these. Who he is is unchangeable, that which does not get lost when age, disease, or circumstances change. Finding out who he is will lead him to the lessons he needs to learn, the work he needs to do. It will lead him to his purpose.

The answers come when men measure themselves by something other than performance, despite what others tell them. They will be incessantly restless until they turn all their woundedness into health, their deformity into beauty, and their embarrassment into laughter.

Male spirituality is always about letting go of a false sense of independence. As youths, men fought for their independence. Dependence meant anxiety, fear, illness, failing, infirmity, and the risk of exploitation. For younger men, dependence meant inferiority. "Stand on your own two feet. Act like a man. Do it yourself. Don't bother with anybody else; you do not need anyone." Through most of their young lives men sought to manage their finances, their households, their careers. To be a man was to be self-sufficient.

Yet they were never fully independent. Men live in a world that is connected to everything that has lived, lives now, and will live. They never were in complete control, despite all of their efforts.

The universal spiritual truth is that no man's life is just about him. There is a far greater story being played out. A man's task in the inward journey is to discover and define his role in that intricate story.

Case Studies: Paul, Michael, Bob, and John

Instead of one extended case study, this section will briefly tell the stories of the spiritual journeys of several men at different stages of life.

Paul is eighty-two years old and describes himself as a religious mutt. He was raised Catholic, practices Buddhist *zazen* and Chinese *Qigong*, and works in an ecumenical organization. He radiates warmth, compassion, wonder, and grace in all he says and does. Yet, he readily confesses that his personal journey has not been easy. He has dealt with the demons of his alcoholism and his compulsive behavior, his workaholism, and his physical infirmities. In recovery now for thirty years, Paul confesses that he has been to his own personal hell and back. He has had many journeys downward to confront his shadow, his false self. Paul will also tell you that without this downward journey, he perhaps never would have found his true self, his essential spiritual nature.

Michael is thirty and tells of his dark night of the soul, when the company he owned went through several audits. A consultant to a major accounting firm reviewed the company books and erroneously concluded that there was fraud, that Michael would be charged, and likely sent to jail. For days, Michael wandered aimlessly through a maze of his fears and terror, only to find out the accountant was totally in error. Michael was guilty of no wrongdoing and his anxiety was ill-founded. The accusation had shaken him to his core and forced him to examine his beliefs and values. What would he be without his career? What was he if not a free man? The terror of that time did not go away easily, and left him seeking a deeper meaning—the answer to the question of who he would be without his job or if he had to forgo his freedom for whatever reason.

Bob, forty-nine, said, "I once thought life was one continuous party, filled with great happiness and very few sorrows. Then my sister died of breast cancer at thirty-six. My son was born with a hearing disability, and my wife was in a serious auto accident that has left her in constant pain. Now I wrestle with the thought that life may just be one sorrow after another. I want to find a balance in my life between joys, which still are many, and sorrows, which seem to come in waves. Why can't life be simple, either happiness or sadness, rather than this living with both?" Bob's spiritual quandary was prompted by that series of tragic events in his immediate family: "How do I live with both sorrow and joy?"

John, twenty-seven, said, "I thought I was doing fine spiritually until my best friend from college, Jack, died at twenty-nine of a heart attack. I became cynical and resentful of people with their seemingly easy lives. My spirituality was rocked, as I was angry with God. How could God allow my friend to die so young, leaving behind a wife and child? It was not until I fully grieved my friend's death that I was able to begin again my conversations with God. Now I see how the outward event of my friend's death was an essential, albeit painful, part of my inward spiritual journey."

These case studies pose another question: Is it necessary to go through such extreme terrors, traumas, and tragedies, to have a spiritual transformation? How can men who have not endured such dramatic experiences undertake their own spiritual journeys?

The following exercises are intended to take the reader through his own spiritual journey, reflecting key issues and questions as steps toward spiritual discovery for men who may or may not have been compelled to examine their lives and spiritual selves as the protagonists in the case studies were. The reader is encouraged to complete each exercise separately in his journal.

Exercise: A Spiritual Inventory

Respond to these statements as honestly as possible. You may experience the following in your daily life. If so, how often? (1 = many times a day, 2 = every day, 3 = most days, 4 = some days, 5 = once in a while, 6 = never or almost never)

1. I feel the presence of something greater than myself (Spirit, Higher Power, God).

2. I experience a connection to all of life.

3. At times (in nature, in community, in worshipful times) I feel a joy that lifts me out of my daily concerns.

4. I find strength and comfort in my faith, my religion, and my spiritual life.

5. I ask for help from my Higher Power, in the midst of my daily activities.

6. I feel guided by my Higher Power in the midst of my daily activities.

7. I feel love for me from something greater than myself.

8. I feel love for me from others.

9. The beauty of creation spiritually touches me.

10. I feel thankful and grateful for my blessings.

11. I feel a selfless caring for others.

12. I desire to be closer to and in union with my Higher Power.

13. In general, I feel close to something greater than myself.

Now, answer these questions:

1. What emotional or physical pain do you still have?

2. How have you transformed your pain?

3. How do you continue to transmit your pain to others or yourself?

4. Who are you today and how does that differ from what you have come to believe you are?

5. How do you fit into the grand scheme of things?

6. Where do you feel significant?

7. What gives you a sense of meaning and purpose in your life?

8. What have been a few of your joys and sorrows in life? How have these joys and sorrows shaped you?

9. Where have you experienced the winning power of love in your life?

10. What control are you still seeking to maintain?

11. Where do you find the courage to change what you can change?

12. What do you need to let go of today?

13. How do you tap into, or find, the serenity to accept what you cannot change?

14. How can you tell the difference between what you can change and what you cannot?

15. When do you feel deep inner peace or harmony?

Five: Work

Work defines most men. When men meet other men one of the first questions they ask is, "What do you do for a living?" They ask this question because, for most of them, their jobs are their identity, the measure of their self-worth, and a central part of their lives. Work connects them to reality. For many, their work is all there is, their job description of life.

The question "What do you do for a living?" also identifies for other men who a man is. It tells them something about that man's status, defining his worth in the world of other men.

Work is also the playing field where men fulfill the honored and respected roles of provider, protector, and producer. If a man chooses to not follow this path in his adulthood, he is often rejected and shamed. These "anti-men" attitudes are widely accepted in the culture and rarely challenged. Men carry a heavy sense of physical responsibility for provision and protection, and this takes a serious toll on men's health and zest for life. Overworking often destroys men's relationships and gives their children less "just being with" time (which is what their children need from them). The amount of time men spend at work seems to be ever-increasing. Men are told that they can easily be replaced and are often taken advantage of in their work environments, creating insecurity and driving them to go beyond what may be emotionally healthy. They work too hard. Eventually they may get to a point in life when they see that they are not just their profit-and-loss statements or career ambitions. They may feel that they have sacrificed too much on work's altar. And they may come to a turning point where they decide to make a change in how they have been living before they have to sacrifice *everything* to their work.

Since the first edition of this book, Version 1.0, there has been a shift in the work life of many men. The Great Recession took its toll on thousands of men, not excluding the authors. Alan was laid off from a center where he had worked for nine years. The "Dark Night of the Soul" gained new meaning for him as he wrestled with the sudden realization that he was dispensable, that he was no longer a part of the company to which he had ascribed his self-worth and value as a man. It took much grieving and soul-searching on his part to accept the loss and be open for new possibilities. The exercises at the end of this chapter were instrumental in that process.

Why do men continue to slog through work that leaves them feeling empty? The promise of a pension somewhere in the future and the security that it offers, the "gold watch" syndrome offering recognition of his endeavor, the gnawing sense that he still does not have enough (whatever "enough" means to him), the feeling that if he worked just a little longer he would finally get that promotion—all contribute to the phenomenon of men continuing to work long after their interest in their work has waned.

So, many men seek to find new joy in their work. To find what brings you joy at work, you may need to turn in another direction, to the inner image of what you were made to be in your work. This may require a period of sobering self-reflection. In his poem, "The Half Turn of Your Face," David Whyte speaks of that moment when you face yourself as you are, yet remember your reflection in the mirror, that which you loved when you were younger and trusted that you would get or achieve everything you wanted. In that moment you make a half turn of your face toward what matters to you now.

The "half turn of your face" is a powerful, compelling concept. It applies so well to finding one's true vocation. It can also be applied on a broader scale to many of the questions explored in this book, such as discovering one's spiritual self or finding meaning in any dimension of one's life. We invite you to think about other ways to make the half turn in the course of your self-discovery.

Case studies: Phillip and Kevin

Phillip made the "half turn of his face" at the age of fifty-one when he ended an eighteen-year career as a minister of a church to try his hand at music writing. Although he continues to support himself as an interim clergyman, his real passion is writing music. He had once been asked, "If someone gave you $100,000 a year and you did not need to worry about making ends meet, what you would do?" Without any hesitation Phillip responded, "Write music." In that moment he began to make the half-turn of his face toward what brought him joy. He was "scared to the core," in David Whyte's words, by the challenges of this half turn of his face, but saw a new reflection of who he was becoming.

Kevin was a forty-five-year-old lawyer with a successful practice in Asheville, North Carolina. He had never been married and had no children. As he looked into the mirror of his life he asked himself, "Is that all there is?" When he made the half turn of his face, the answer to his question was, "No, I want to give back to society in a different way. I want to work in the helping professions." He left his law practice and returned to school for a degree in social work. He now works in a shelter for homeless men. He feels a new sense of significance, not in material terms but in the legacy of compassion he is leaving behind in the lives of the men he helps.

Perhaps it is time to change your outlook on work, to find what fulfills your inner needs.

Downshifting

Here are other stories men tell about how they view work. Tom says, "I am bored in my job. But here I am, fifty-two, and I'll be working into my late sixties. I have a young son who will be entering college when I am sixty-five years old. Retirement? Not for a long time."

Carl, fifty-four, says, "I am earning a million dollars a year as a corporate president. I hate my job, but I am scared to death of losing it. If I do, I will not be able to live in the manner to which my family and I have grown accustomed."

Stanley says, "I have worked most of my life. It is not that I don't want to work any longer, I just don't want to work as hard."

Some men want to downshift, to work fewer hours or with less responsibility or pressure. Here are steps you can take to change your work pattern if you are thinking of downshifting:

- Keep lunchtime personal.
- Avoid weekend business travel.
- Make firm personal appointments.
- Set reasonable deadlines. Set stop times.
- Negotiate extra vacation time. Arrange flextime.
- Go part-time.
- Make a lateral or downward move.
- Decline a promotion.
- Telecommute.
- Take early or gradual retirement.

Case Study: Bruce

Bruce was a successful electrician with a solid book of business. He'd learned the electrical trade after high school and started his own business in his twenties. He was financially successful, happily married, and his children were grown. Yet Bruce knew there was more to life than money in the bank and saving for retirement. At fifty-eight, Bruce decided he needed to downshift, to work less and put in fewer hours. He met with his accountant and found a way to cash in and access his retirement funds early. He sold his business and bought a house in the Mexican mountains. From there he did electrical contracting jobs in Mexico and the United States. As a hedge against his fear of not having enough, he opened a small business in Boulder, Colorado, and lived half of the year in Mexico and the other half in Colorado. Bruce soon learned that he did not need the Colorado business and that his life was very full in Mexico. He "retired" to work only in Mexico.

Bruce downshifted in two steps from a full-time business to more relaxed work. Bruce now picks and chooses the work that gives him energy and passion. He has been an inspiration to many.

Downshifting does not necessarily mean that you stop working entirely; rather, it means that you focus on what you want to do and how you want to do it, not just what you need to do.

Exercise: The Role of Work in Your Life

Answer these questions:

1. How do you introduce yourself at a party?
2. What is the lure of work for you?
3. What has work become for you?
4. What is the toll of today's workplace on you?
5. What would you do if you did not have to work? If you were given your salary for a year and were able to take a sabbatical, what would you do? Most importantly, what questions would you want answered during your sabbatical?
6. Have you become your work?
7. Is work an escape from other parts of your life, into a world under your control?
8. Do you feel as if you have climbed the ladder of success only to realize that the ladder is leaning against the wrong building?
9. Do you sometimes feel lost at work? Have you experienced an internal sticker shock, seeing that the price you paid for career advancement was your vitality, passion, and commitments?

Exercise: Workplace Robbers

Review the following list of workplace robbers and ask yourself whether any of them are issues or concerns for you at work.

Competitive pressures:

Do you feel you have to do more to gain someone's approval, or because someone else is there behind you desiring your job?

The corporate culture:

Do you put in extra hours on evenings, weekends, or holidays because your colleagues do? Do you feel as if you have to do more with less?

The need to "make the numbers":

Do you feel pressured to meet sales quotas or profit benchmarks, to do better? Do you feel the pressure to serve more people?

Rapid change:

Are you running as fast as you can but never able to keep up with the pace of change?

Overwhelming work burdens:

Is there too much to do and not enough time to do it? What has work become for you? Are you rusted out at work? Have you lost the fire and passion you once had?

Exercise: Finding Fulfilling Work

Answer the following questions:

1. What were you created to be in life?
2. Is what you are currently doing that thing for which you were created?
3. What aspects of your current work fulfill your "destiny"?
4. What can you bring into your work that enlivens and perhaps even scares you a little?

✐ Exercise: The Circle Game

Draw a large circle on half a page in your journal. In that circle write down the qualities you can express in your current work. For example, it might be your creativity, your skills, your passion and compassion, the joys and problems of working with people, etc.

Below the circle write the qualities you would like to express in life. These may be qualities such as expressing love, making an impact on others, being a change agent, leaving a record of your creativity, having a sense of peace, quiet, and joy, participating in a spiritual journey to serenity, finding more leisure time, etc.

Which of these qualities can be expressed in your current work? Write them inside the circle at the top. Which qualities cannot be expressed in your current work environment? Write these qualities outside the circle. As you look over what is inside and outside the circle, mark the three items that are most important to you at this point in your life. How can you bring into your work those items outside the circle that are most important to you? The essence of work should be to find what you truly love to do. When these qualities cannot be brought into your work, you need to find a way to make them part of your life as a whole.

✐ Exercise: Finding Your Calling

In the case studies earlier in this chapter, Philip, Kevin, and Bruce not only heard the drum of their calling but were able to manage the monetary costs of the career change foretold by the beat. For others, like Carl and Tom, the chronic pain of their chosen careers was becoming unbearable, with no relief in sight. How do we find our calling, especially if it has been buried under heaps of activities over time? One way to hear that drum is to conduct a job interview of ourselves.

First, finding your heartbeat begins in stillness. Get away from the chatter around you and retreat to aloneness, where you can listen to the voice of your soul that says, "Do this. This is what you were meant to be." Bubbling up from deep within you, listen to the stillness that calls you back to your dreams.

Listen to the yearnings that sneak up on you in subtle ways. You may be watching a movie and something grabs you, saying, "Pay attention to this. This is important." Figure out what this calling will cost you and people in your life. Ask yourself what you are willing to pay in time, money, and emotions to respond to this calling.

Now answer these questions in your journal:

1. What do you feel called to do at this stage of your life? What gives you a sense of wholeness in life? (When you find it, then that is likely your calling.)

2. What parts of you have gone undeveloped or underdeveloped in your life and work thus far? (It is those parts of you that have been lost in the shadows that may now be seeking light.)

3. What is still waiting to be born in you?

4. What would be incomplete in your life if you never did this one thing?

Exercise: Number Your Days— Having a Sense of Wonder and Gratitude

Building on the previous exercises, let's take this experience of self-exploration to another level. This exercise extends and enlarges the inquiry, putting work in the broader context of life satisfaction.

List the things that have given you the greatest joy in life. Focus on each of the people and joyful events in each period of your life.

List the times you have felt awe and the circumstances that brought that about.

Make this week, month, or year a celebration of your life by making a pilgrimage to a significant place of joy in your life. Plan a special day to celebrate your life. Help someone else celebrate the joys of their life story. Put together an album of photos and mementos of joyous and wondrous times in your life.

Visit and talk with people from your past who gave you perspective on different aspects of your life. Celebrate your roots by attending an ethnic festival. Read poetry or prose from your heritage. Listen to its music.

List the conflicts of your life that have taught you something important. Conduct an internal dialogue with the ones that seem most significant. Give yourself a day of fun, a time of wonder and joy.

Six: Money

What is it about men and money? It is generally the last frontier we men will ever cross or talk about with others. Men talk about money in code. "So, what do you do for a living?" works as a measuring stick to determine indirectly what a man earns. If a man tells you he is a laborer or a CEO, you generally have some idea what he is worth, and how much he makes.

Money means many things to men: power, possessions, prestige, perks, and possibilities. The specter of *not* having money, and therefore *not* having power, possessions, etc. drives men to work and overwork. They worry about having enough money to provide for and respond to their families' needs and/or maintain their chosen lifestyles.

Work and money are interwoven and play significant roles in the lives of many men, so it is important to address both of these issues.

Money brings men alive, giving meaning to what they do. For many, money is all there is.

Money may mean that men are able to buy the things that they and their families desire, or think they desire. Until recently, men identified their needs and then saved money until they could make the purchases. This gave work a sense of meaning. Work may not have been particularly satisfying, but at least it had an identifiable purpose that was likely appreciated at home, in the workplace, or in society as a whole. Today, seeking instant gratification of our desires, we buy on credit. As a result, money is detached from the item initially purchased and becomes merely a way of paying off credit card debt. Today, it often feels like a never-ending cycle of work and spending: the mortgage, kids' college education, saving for retirement, our "toys," and, for some, child support or alimony.

Since 2008 many men have had to readjust their financial goals and aspirations. As the era of excess, exemplified by material goods, from Hummers to McMansions, came to a grinding halt, paying for that consumption became impossible. Millions have lost homes and filed personal bankruptcy. Many of these bankrupts, these former homeowners—men no longer able to identify themselves by their professions—have become "used-to-bes." The struggle for reemployment, the opportunity to step back on the ladder, has, thus far, been unattainable for many.

For countless others, the wars in Iraq and Afghanistan became their focus as they served their country. As the wars wind down, those returning servicemen (and women) are finding fewer and fewer job opportunities as they return to their hometowns.

Affluenza

Some men (and women) suffer from a common ailment: affluenza. We have too much, and yet want more. Simply defined, affluenza is the name for a dysfunctional relationship with or pursuit of money/wealth. Globally, it is a backup in the flow of money resulting in a polarization of the classes and a loss of economic and emotional balance. We can see the symptoms of affluenza throughout our culture: in those around us who have wealth, in those who are pursuing wealth, and in varying degrees within ourselves.

A clinical definition is as follows:

The collective addiction, character flaws, psychological wounds, neuroses, and behavioral disorders caused or exacerbated by the presence of or desire for money/wealth. In corporations and businesses it manifests as a loss of personal and professional productivity, high turnover rate among CEOs and employees, and an increase in sick days.

In individuals it takes the form of a dysfunctional or unhealthy relationship with money, regardless of one's socioeconomic level. It manifests as behaviors resulting from a preoccupation with—or imbalance around—the money in our lives.

The psychological dysfunctions of affluenza within the family are generational; they are frequently passed from parent to child. The symptoms of affluenza are:

- Loss of personal and professional productivity
- Loss of motivation
- Inability to delay gratification or tolerate frustration
- False sense of entitlement
- Low self-esteem

- Low self-worth
- Loss of self-confidence
- Preoccupation with externals
- Depression
- Self-absorption
- High regard for outer self/low regard for inner self; "survivor's" guilt/shame
- Sudden wealth syndrome
- Sudden poverty syndrome
- Workaholism
- Addiction
- Other compulsive-addictive behaviors, e.g., rampant materialism and consumerism

The psychological dynamics of affluenza are more complex and more harmful than one popularized definition of affluenza as merely "a rich person's disease" would have it. People across all socioeconomic levels buy into the overriding value our culture places on money, and the assumption that money solves all problems. Thus, denial of money-related difficulties is supported by society, and many sufferers of affluenza hesitate to seek help.

Affluenza can be successfully overcome. With personal insight into the potentially crippling effects that the obsession with money can have on every aspect of our lives—professionally and personally—we can begin to create our own monetary intentions and employ our money in more appropriate ways. We can learn how to create emotional balance in financial matters in the work environment, resulting in a more successful business and, most importantly, a more balanced and successful lifestyle.

Case Studies: Roger, Carl, and Jim

This section will provide vignettes of several men to illustrate how they look at money.

Roger is the CEO of a Fortune 500 company. His estimated income in 1990 was 26 million dollars, not bad for a man who barely finished college and inherited his company from his father. He lived in a mansion in Greenwich, Connecticut, and flew weekly in the corporate jet to his "castle" home in Florida, which stretched from the Atlantic Ocean to the Intracoastal Waterway.

One night one of the authors, David, was visiting Roger and his wife as a guest in their Florida home. After a delicious meal prepared by a five-star chef, they relaxed in their "den" and retired early. Awakened around midnight by noise in the kitchen, David went downstairs to see what was going on. There in the kitchen, Roger and his wife were going over their checkbook, paying bills. David said to Roger's wife, Jean, "Why are you doing that, Jean? You could hire a room full of accountants to do your checkbook." Jean responded, "We don't trust anyone else with our personal checkbook." David was astonished and retired to bed, having seen that money does not necessarily bring peace of mind.

A second case is Carl, an executive vice president of another Fortune 500 company. He was earning over one million dollars a year, not counting stock options. One year the business was undergoing major financial problems and the board of directors was exploring changes in their management structure. Carl was worried he'd lose his job. In a conversation, Carl expressed his anxiety about being out of work.

Carl said, "I am worried I will lose my job. I am fifty years old with a huge mortgage and a family to support. Who will hire me?" When asked about the source of his anxiety, Carl's response was, "If I should lose my job I might not be able to provide the lifestyle my wife and family are accustomed to." With a net worth of tens of millions, he was fearful that he'd have to cut back his spending. Carl and his family truly suffered from "affluenza."

Jim is a laborer, getting by on $35,000 a year. His wife works as a maid in a hotel, and their combined annual income barely exceeds $50,000, from which they have to pay their mortgage, living expenses, and looming college tuition bills for their two children. Despite all this, Jim and his wife Sue were contented with their life and felt little fear about the loss of their income.

Although work was spotty for Jim, he rested at night with the assurance that "everything will be okay." Jim thought, "We have little, yet we know all will be well. We will not be out on the street. There is food on the table, we are a closely knit family, we love each other dearly, and life is good."

These three men have very different attitudes about money, net worth, and security. The point is not that accumulation of wealth is a bad thing, or that poverty or living close to the poverty line is to be desired. Instead, happiness is in the eyes of the beholder. The key question every man needs to ask himself is, "How much would I be worth if I lost all of my money?" The answer to that question might determine one's level of peace, anxiety, security, and happiness. After all, it is not happy (or wealthy) people who are grateful but grateful people who are happy.

Do you find yourself often reflecting on your net worth and assets? Do you keep mental tally sheets of what you have accumulated so far? Do you hire a financial planner to assure you that there is enough for the future? The following exercises may illuminate your position on money.

✎ Exercise: Do You Have Affluenza?

Diagnose yourself using the key below.

1. I'm willing to pay more for a t-shirt if it has a cool corporate logo on it.

2. I believe that if I buy the expensive suit, the promotion will come.

3. I have a tie collection Donald Trump would envy.

4. When I'm cold, I take my clothes off and turn up the heat.

5. I'm willing to work forty years at a job I hate so I can buy lots of stuff.

6. When I'm feeling down, I like to go on eBay and treat myself.

7. I want or have a sport utility vehicle, although I rarely drive in conditions that warrant having one.

8. I usually make just the minimum payment on my credit cards.

9. I'd rather be golfing right now.

10. I believe that whoever dies with the most toys wins.

11. Most of the things my friends/family and I enjoy doing together are free.

12. I don't measure my self-worth (or that of others) by what I own.

13. I know how to pinch a dollar until it screams.

14. I worry about the effects of advertising on children.

15. To get to work, I carpool, ride my bike, or use public transportation.

For questions one through ten, give yourself two points for true and one point for false. For questions eleven through fourteen, give yourself zero points for true and two points for false.

If you scored:

Ten to fifteen: No dangerous signs of affluenza at this time.

Sixteen to twenty-two: Warning—you have mild affluenza.

Twenty-three to thirty: Cut up your credit cards and call a doctor immediately!

Exercise: Your Spiritual Financial Journey

Step One

Imagine yourself setting out on a journey. During this journey, you are in search of the qualities in your life that you still want to find. What "lands and destinations" do you seek to visit? Think about both geographic and life milestones as destinations for yourself. For example, are there places in the world you want to see? Are there adventures you still wish to experience? What areas of significance and meaning do you still wish to have in your world? Are there emotional, physical, and social events or experiences you still want to have in your life's journey? Where would you still like to go in your career and profession?

Write down the work "destinations" where you still wish to go, the journey you still want to take in your life.

Step Two

What do you need for the journey? How much money do you really need to enjoy the journey? What would you need to take along on this trip? Personal possessions, music to listen to, books to read, people you wish to be with, sacred objects, etc.? What other items would you bring, such as social, emotional, and spiritual qualities? List at least fourteen items.

Step Three

Follow the old rule in packing for a trip: take what you have packed and cut that in half. You have probably packed too much already. You have more than you will ever need for your life's journey. Cut the above list in half, down to no more than seven items.

Step Four:

Now cut the list again, this time down to three items. What are the three most important items you will need for your journey?

Those are probably all you will need for the rest of your life's journey in work. This may be a difficult and painful exercise, casting off the power, possessions, and work prestige you have accumulated so far. But in all likelihood you do not need these anymore. In fact, they may be an impediment to your life's journey at work. Your preoccupation with these items can weigh you down.

Seven: Men and Their Children

The father-child bond, especially the father-son bond, may be the most significant relationship in a man's life. It is essential that you explore this relationship on your journey, because many men carry strong feelings both about their own fathers and about their role as fathers to their children. Even if a man has no biological children of his own, he may be a stepfather, godfather, or "chosen father" to someone else's children, he may be thinking of one day being a father, or he may have feelings about what it might be like to be a father. It is essential for a man to understand the role that his own father has played in his life. If he has a child, it is important to explore how to be a spiritual father and how to be a healthy parent.

First, it is important to acknowledge the many variations of the father-child relationship: single fathers, stepfathers, fathers with multiple families, gay fathers, and so forth. So we do not want to imply that fathering involves only the traditional father-child relationship.

One of the beauties of life today is that there does not seem to be a uniform pattern to fit all men. They are making it up as they go along.

A man can help his sons and daughters by sharing his inner life with them, by being open about his thoughts, feelings, dreams, and hurts. As a way of preparing his sons for manhood, a man can telecast the journey he has been through to inform and coach his sons through their eventual journey. If a man is in recovery from addiction, this is especially important because we know addiction runs in families.

When a man's children get to different stages of their lives, they likely will remember the stories of their father's hurts and how he wrestled with them. Perhaps they will consult with their father for guidance through their own journeys. If a man's sons received good masculine energy from their father, or another positive male model, as they grew up, they likely will not reject guidance when they are grown. A positive male figure can teach a boy how to be a man in a healthy, balanced way.

Most importantly, a son needs to believe that his father respects and admires him. He wants his dad to be proud of him. As he grows into adulthood, a father's pride may seem patronizing if a foundation of appreciation and praise was not laid in childhood. What a boy needs all along is not just his parents' approval (which we hope most boys receive), but also adult respect and honest admiration. The honoring of the boy is what eventually invites him into the club of men. This invitation lets him know that he is his father's equal.

To be a mature father, a man can also teach his sons and daughters lessons or virtues such as self-possession, truthfulness, responsibility, closure, and challenge.

Self-possession is the virtue of self-knowledge. It is the ability to be in touch with one's center, feelings, and motives. A self-possessed man has self-knowledge and awareness. He knows (as well as any of us realistically can) where he is coming from and where he is going. He seeks the well-being of others and not simply what he wants for himself.

The second virtue is truthfulness, which is knowledge of reality. It is one's ability to see clearly what is going on in the world. Truthfulness means being able to name truth. This virtue presupposes that a man is objective and detached from the situation he is viewing. It means that he has balanced judgment and does not project his own biases and prejudices onto the situation. Sometimes a man has to be truthful about things with which he is emotionally involved. This can be difficult and requires wisdom and maturity.

The third virtue, responsibility, is the opposite of passivity. Another term for this might be *initiative*. A responsible father does not need to be told what to do; he does it and assumes responsibility for his actions. This does not mean "shooting from the hip" or being a "ready, fire, aim" guy. It means taking appropriate action when needed.

Closure, the fourth virtue, is the virtue needed when a decision must be made. It is an essential element of responsible decision-making.

Finally, challenge is the virtue that might be called "tough love." If forgiveness is the ability to let go of hurts, then challenge is the ability to risk hurting. This is not negative or destructive action, but action always guided by love. It requires forthrightness. Challenge means being willing to risk argument, misunderstanding, and disagreement—being willing to stick your neck out for a person or a value in which you believe.

Today many children live with their parents long after they are grown because they cannot afford to live anywhere else. This offers a new opportunity for fathers to learn how to nurture their children. But fathers have to be willing to suspend decades of cultural conditioning and learn how to be nurturers as well as providers if they want to take advantage of this opportunity. They will have to learn the language of the heart, to feel what a child feels and to acknowledge the truth of those feelings—without acting on the urge to correct, punish, or reward. Today, younger fathers are making great strides in learning how to nurture their children and are deriving personal benefits from these life changes. Even a man who fathers a baby late in life can transform his behavior.

Fatherhood has as much of an influence on mental and physical health as career achievement does. Fathers who are highly invested in their work but who also care about their children and spend significant time with them can still have an important effect on the emotional well-being of their children, and, by extension, on their own emotional well-being. The most promising direction for redefining masculinity lies in reinventing fatherhood. Most of the reinvented fathers are now in their twenties and thirties, but not all. Some are "start-over" dads in their late forties and fifties, raising second families.

They could not look to their dads as role models for nurturing. Most were taught to separate quickly from their parents and move away. No doubt many men today did not have fathers who were models of caring, emotional expressiveness, and involvement with their children. Some of these men, who now have an opportunity to parent a second family, choose to make different decisions about childrearing than they did with their first children, and seek to bring more warmth and gentleness into their parenting this time around.

These generational contrasts are valid up to a point, but as with any generalization, there are exceptions. Many men who came of age in the 1960s were part of a generation that also separated quickly from parents and moved away, in part because they were trying to live by different values from those of their parents, and thus could not identify closely with their fathers. But one expression of their generation's idealism was to try to be parents in different ways—to be more available, "soft," and nurturing—and thereby avoid the kinds of conflicts they had had with their parents.

Breaking down gender roles, with fathers more actively present in childrearing and sharing both the burden and the positive experience more equally with mothers, was part of this cultural evolution. There are many men, now in their fifties and sixties, who were that kind of father—and not just the second time around, but also in their thirties and perhaps their twenties (although many baby boomers had children late, so it is likely that they were more mature and thoughtful when they began as parents). On a recent radio program about "Generation Y" (the children of baby boomers), it was observed that these young people often regard their parents as "good friends." That's one reason (besides economic necessity) why these children, more often than not, live with their parents than did the young adults of the sixties. So some credit must be given to the sixties and seventies counterculture for changing values and practices in parenting.

Fathers play critical roles in the lives of their children:

1. Fathers can provide additional nurturing that is critical in early development of children. Although nurturing is commonly associated with the mother's role, fathers, too, need to nurture their children through expressions of love and caring.

2. Fathers can be role models. Children need positive male role models whom they can admire and emulate.

3. Fathers initiate boys into manhood. Traditionally this initiation happened through an experience of the wonders of nature and by

the boy facing his frailties and limitations. Vision quests and bar mitzvahs were traditional initiation rites. Initiation moves a young man from a natural self-centeredness to a more mature, healthy inclusion of others. This becomes a critical factor in helping to ensure success later in life. A man should ask himself how he is initiating his son(s) into manhood.

4. Fathers can be mentors. Mentoring continues the process by which a young man grows and matures. As a mentor the father teaches the son how to be a productive member of the community and society. The mentor provides advice, sponsorship, and guidance.

5. Fathers can be elders. The older father can teach the boy-turned-man the wisdom learned through the ages. This wisdom involves a shift from the outside to the inside, from the physical to the spiritual, and from egocentricity to community-centeredness.

You may work overtime or work two jobs to make ends meet. One day you wake up and the children have cars and are spending their evenings and weekends away from the home. Then the kids get jobs or go to college. Nature seems to play a mean trick on you: the years when your children are growing are your most financially productive years. These are the years of ascent. Yet, by the time you realize that this lifestyle is taking a toll on you and your family, it is often too late. Your children are teens and have active lives of their own or do not desire to spend time with their "boring parents." A "family vacation" with teenagers is an oxymoron. The time for healthy family vacations may be over before it begins for you and your family. You may realize you have spent all of these years doing what you were told to do to win your father's and family's respect, but in the process have lost precious time with your children and spouse. It is time you can never fully reclaim. You may feel a void as you realize that, while dedicating your life to a successful career and being a good provider for your family, you have missed out on the deeper, more rewarding aspects of your life and parenting.

What do you need to do today to find time in your life for your children? What activities would they enjoy doing with you? What would you like to do with them? Is it time to change your priorities in life, to reorganize your life to become the father you long to be?

Exercise: What Kind of Father Are You?

It is important for men to take an inventory of our role as a father up until now, whether our children are young or old, male or female. Answer the following questions in your journal:

1. In what ways were you involved in your children's birth?

2. Do you feel that you matter to your children? In what ways?

3. When your children were born, what kind of father did you want to be? Have you been that kind of father to them?

4. How much alone time do (did) you spend with your children?

5. What rituals did (do) you have with your kids?

6. What was (is) your policy on physical punishment of your children?

7. In what ways are you a domineering father?

8. Are you sensitive to gender-related issues with your children?

9. Do you and your spouse communicate at cross-purposes with your children?

10. Do you draw the kids in as allies in family arguments?

Exercise: The Father You Long To Be

What kind of father do you long to be? In your journal answer the following:

- Describe the qualities of the father you long to be (emotional, physical, social, and spiritual).

- What is your reaction to the following lessons you might pass on to your children?

  - How to win and how to lose with dignity, and how to play the games of life without always having to win

  - How to be a team player

  - How to interact with women and with other men

  - How to surrender, to be spiritual, to pray

  - How to guide, teach, and lead

  - How to commit to something, such as how to love and receive love

  - How to like oneself, to be appropriately proud of oneself

  - How to respect self, others, the environment

  - How to experience and express one's feelings appropriately

  - How to touch appropriately

  - How to value one's own body

  - How to care, to have hope, and to help others with wisdom

  - How to find and use power respectfully

  - How to value work appropriately, to have a vocation as well as an avocation

  - How to laugh, cry, think, and follow through with whatever has to be done

  - How to end relationships, when necessary, in a careful and caring manner

This inventory has described the father you are, have been, or long to be, as you perceive yourself. The next step is to ask yourself these questions:

- How do you live out these values with your children? How do you make your "father love" accessible to your children?

- What kind of father do you now want to be to your children?

- How can you add more time with your children, regardless of what age they may be?

- What spiritual wisdom have you learned so far in your life that you want to pass on to your children?

- How can you find the time and opportunities to pass this spiritual wisdom on to them?

- How can you be a wise elder to your children?

- If in recovery, how has your addiction interfered with or affected your role as a father to your children? To children other than your own?

- How can you now teach your children about self-possession, truthfulness, responsibility, closure, and challenge? What do you want to say to them about these virtues, based on your own experiences so far in life?

- What kind of help do you need to be the father you want to be?

- What is your Achilles' heel as a father? It could be your temper, impatience, arrogance, or ignorance about children, adolescents, or young adults, or something else entirely.

Exercise: Action Steps You Can Take

Next, it is time to act. How can you take the following steps with your children? Write down the action(s) you are prepared to take now to change your relationship with your children.

Step One

The first step is to review your time commitments with your children. Despite all of the changing images of fatherhood discussed previously, even today you may return home long after your young children are in bed. Even if your children are still awake when you get home, you may close yourself off by tuning into TV, alcohol, or other numbing behaviors. You may take business trips away from the family for days and weeks at a time. What are you willing to change in this regard?

Step Two

Is it time for you to do something spiritually refreshing with your children? Perhaps you need to offer refreshing spiritual experiences to your children and yourself. You cannot give much to your children when you are running on empty.

Here are some hints to refresh your spiritual life with your children:

- Find a faith community or spiritual activity that you and your children can share. What would work for you and your children?

- Share spiritually-oriented books with your children. This can be as simple as reading stories from books such as *Chicken Soup for the Soul* to more profound spiritual writing. Share the poetry of Hafiz or Rumi. Read Annie Dillard or Annie Lamont, who speak of their lives' journeys. Read books with your sons like Richard Rohr's *The Wild Man's Journey*. What would you and your children enjoy reading together?

- Go for a walk together in nature. Talk about nature's wonders, the mysteries of creation, the sounds of silence one finds in the forest or mountains, the sense of awe and wonder that nature brings. Talk about your prior experiences in nature, your spiritual yearning for something greater than yourself, or your sense of majesty when confronted by the magnitude of creation. How can you make this happen in your life as a parent?

- Talk with your children, especially when they are teenagers or older, about your own experience of powerlessness and the wounds and hurts in your life. Be vulnerable with your children. Tell on yourself; share stories of your life experience. What can you do today to begin the conversation anew with your children?

- What activities do you really enjoy that you could share with your children, such as hiking, biking, fishing, or skiing? Maybe these activities were shared in the past but haven't been for some time. Which ones could you begin to engage in today?

Step Three

Spend time with other fathers. Talk with them about the fathers they long to be. You will learn that you are not alone on this journey. With what other men in your life can you share your interests and concerns as a father?

Exercise: Write an Ethical Will

Much as a man would write a will of his goods and possessions, a man can write a will that reflects the ethical, moral, and spiritual teachings and principles he wishes to leave his children. Answering the following questions will help you to write an ethical will to your children, regardless of their ages.

1. What would you leave behind in the hearts and minds of each of your children?

2. Would you leave different principles for your son(s) than your daughter(s)? How would they differ?

3. What lessons have you learned in life that you'd like your children to know?

You need not give the ethical will to your children at this time. That depends on their ages. If they are teenagers or adults you may wish to sit down with each of them and go over what you wrote in your ethical will.

Section II Notes

1. George E. Vaillant, *Aging Well: Surprising Guideposts to a Happier Life from the Landmark Harvard Study of Adult Development* (New York: Little, Brown and Company, 2002).

2. Gail Sheehy, *Understanding Men's Passages: Discovering the New Map of Men's Lives* (New York: Ballantine Books, 1999).

3. Maria Kubin et al., "Epidemiology of erectile dysfunction," *International Journal of Impotence Research*, volume 15, number 1, (2003) pp. 63–71.

4. Ibid.

5. Sharon Wegscheider-Cruse and Joseph Cruse, *Understanding Co-Dependency* (Deerfield Beach: Health Communications, Inc., 1990).

6. Lucia Capacchione, *Recovery of Your Inner Child: The Highly Acclaimed Method for Liberating Your Inner Self* (New York: Touchstone, 1991).

7. Jennifer Schneider and Robert Weiss, *Cybersex Exposed: Simple Fantasy or Obsession?* (Center City: Hazelden, 2001), p. 7.

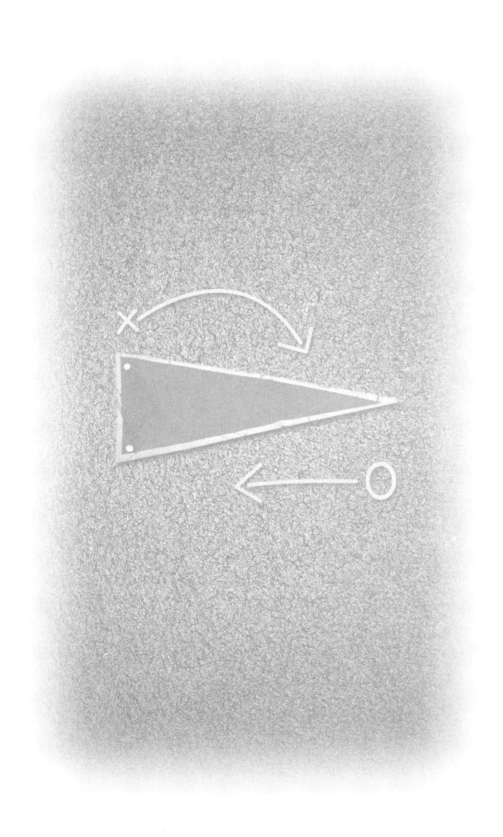

Section III: Helping Men/Healing Men

One: The Importance and Challenges of Gender-Specific Treatment

There are several advantages of male clinicians working in all-male settings. Some well-known treatment centers place men in all-male groups with only male counselors and women in all-female groups with only female counselors. It has been the experience of these programs that all-male groups with only male counselors (and vice versa for the female clients), are a more effective way of structuring treatment. But, whether the treatment is administered by men, for men, or whether women counselors are treating men, there are compelling reasons to have all-male treatment groups.

Generally speaking, men are task- and goal-oriented and seek autonomy. A process that is tailored to support and reflect men's quest for autonomy helps men to heal. For most male substance-abuse clients, being in an all-male, homogeneous group presents some distinct advantages that are not available in mixed gender groups. All-male groups offer familiar terrain at a time when a man may feel particularly alienated. Although men often function in the public sphere, surrounded by work associates, and often report a large number of "buddies" or casual friends—men, particularly substance-dependent men, live lives of marked emotional isolation. Brehm found that men tend to have friendships characterized by "activity sharing" (e.g., hunting, working on a car, playing cards), whereas women are more likely to have friendships characterized by interpersonal intimacy and disclosure of feelings.[1] Men generally prefer "side-by-side" relationships, whereas women prefer "face-to-face" relationships.

Because men lead these emotionally isolated lives, many men find that therapy/support groups offer immense potential for interpersonal communication and connectedness and recognition of common struggles. Yalom spoke of the importance of universality in groups, the awareness that we are all in the same boat together.[2] Anecdotal research indicates that men also form bonds with other men faster, are more self-disclosing, and sense a greater kinship and brotherhood with other men when women are not present. Farrell noted a tendency of men to practice "self-listening," whereby a man listens to a conversation, not to take in or genuinely appreciate what another man is saying, but only to be able to jump in and discuss his own experiences.[3] Men engage in "report talk," not "rapport talk."[4] The group, as a social microcosm, is abundant with opportunities for men to experience the consequences of their communication style. When encouraged to experiment with alternatives, men can become far more effective in the interpersonal realm.

All-male groups instill hope through listening to the testimonies of other men. This is where some of the power of twelve-step groups lies; men have a chance to listen to other personal stories and can find expectancy and hope in those stories. They provide a major source of incentive and demystification for men who might otherwise see counseling as a threatening or emasculating process. Group work further aids in the discovery of emotional connections. Although men can share deep and intense feelings and are capable of interpersonal connections, they typically interact intensely only when fighting or competing. Strong emotions expressed by one group member generate considerable emotional resonance with other group members in other men, heightening the intensity of the change process. Many men in groups are amazed to realize the strength of the feelings they have suppressed.

Furthermore, male-specific groups aid in overcoming men's frequent dependence on women to talk for them, as was the case with Chris in Chapter Three. Because men limit emotional expressiveness and intimacy with other men, they tend to become dependent on women to express their emotions for them, and they may experience their emotions vicariously through them. And, although men often rely on women to carry their emotions in a mixed gender therapy group, they can end up treating the women in the group differently by either placating or pandering to them, further entrenching old, negative patterns of treating women. Because men have allowed themselves to become so dependent on women for social facilitation, nurturance, and validation, the all-male therapy/support group offers a valuable corrective emotional experience, as men learn together to trust and value intimate male friendships and express their own emotions without female influence.

Men are traditionally extremely wary of personal revelations, feeling that private admissions could cause them to be seen in a negative light. Individual counseling further exacerbates this inhibition, given the power differential between client and therapist. This feeling can be especially strong if the counselor is a woman. The all-male group provides a potent environment to counter this antitherapeutic pattern, so common among men in individual therapy, by encouraging participative self-disclosure.

Male gender role socialization can contribute to a tendency for men to deny, misperceive, and minimize their need for assistance, particularly when that assistance is for biological, medical, or behavioral problems. For some men, seeking out a professional helper threatens their sense of masculinity. Since men are taught to ignore physical and psychic pain, they may see their distress as an inability to manage their own problems. It may reflect a sense of low self-esteem, incompetence, a perceived loss of autonomy, or a fear of dependence on others for help.

As they do with most healthcare problems, men tend to seek treatment later in the addictive process than their female counterparts. Even when they do seek help, men may do so only in response to some external pressure, such as a DUI, threat of job loss, etc., and may deny or minimize the severity of the issue. Given this reluctance to seek assistance, it is important that healthcare professionals maximize whatever opportunity they have to fully evaluate a man's condition and to engage him in a helping relationship. Given that the quality of the therapeutic alliance has been found to be the single most important predictor of treatment outcome, the rapid establishment of a therapeutic relationship with a male client cannot be overemphasized.

Clinicians might acknowledge that substance-abusing men can be aggressive, often commit property crimes, and may present in a state of acute intoxication. As a result, when men are seen for substance abuse assessment, the physical setting and clinical procedures must allow for effective management of aggressive behavior, prevention of theft (particularly if cash or medications are kept on-site), and effective management of acute intoxication.

In sum, because male socialization emphasizes independence, emotional stoicism, isolation, and maintaining "power over" in relationships, male resistance to counseling should be anticipated, understood, and respected. An effective tool for dealing with this socialization process is group work, which can propel men into a journey that will profoundly alter their lives.

The Challenges

The 70/70 Percent Rule: A Female-Dominated Profession

Approximately 70 percent of the clients in addiction treatment programs in America are men. Although the majority of management personnel in treatment programs are men, 57–60 percent of the counselors in addiction treatment programs are women; this figure increases when traditionally female-dominant professions such as nurses, aids, educators, social workers, and social service workers are included. Approximately 70 percent of new counselors entering the addiction field are female.

Counselors need gender-oriented training. The addiction counseling profession will not remedy the gender imbalance in treatment until salaries are on par with similar professions and society's attitude about men in care-providing positions changes. Therefore, given the fact that the preponderance of counselors in the field will likely, for some time, remain female, we must address how to best work with men.

Why are these professions female-dominated? The issue is in part about money. The average salary for an addiction counselor in America in 2012 was in the mid-$40,000s. The salary for a full-time counselor ranged from $37,000–$64,000. More women are entering the field later in life as a second career, after they have raised their children, and often to provide a second income for the family.

These data raise profound questions about how addiction treatment is delivered in America, especially for men. If the majority of the patients are male and the majority of the care providers are female, there may be a need to address the specific issues of men in treatment. This means that gender-sensitive treatment for men and for women is needed in order to ensure the delivery of the most responsive and effective therapy possible.

Women as Clinicians in All-Male Settings

Given the preponderance of female counselors, how can the treatment experience be maximized for men? In some respects, female clinicians do play a beneficial role for male clients. Research indicates that men report matters about their family of origin more readily to female counselors than to male counselors.[5] Men are generally more comfortable with women counselors when discussing affective issues. For their part, female counselors tend to be process-oriented rather than task-oriented. This is advantageous for some men, who otherwise might readily avoid dealing with their emotions by remaining task-oriented in therapy.

There are, on the other hand, some problems for women working as clinicians in all-male settings. First, some men may see their male counselors (if there are any in the agency) as the "real therapists," having the "real power" in the organization. Some men have difficulty "hearing" their female counselors, which likely has to do with differences between how men and women communicate.[6] Some men may not be accustomed to communicating openly with women. Moreover, a female counselor cannot provide a positive male role model for a male client simply because she is not a man.

There may be a clash of styles between female clinicians and male clinicians or clients. "Masculine" is often thought to suggest "didactic, scientific, detached, noncommittal" qualities. "Feminine" may be thought to mean "collaborative, noncompetitive, and nurturing." This stereotyping of behavior can be destructive to the therapeutic process.

Some male clients may view the nurturing offered by a female clinician as "smothering." Female clinicians can project their own antagonism toward men onto their male clients.

Attachment theory holds that a female clinician working in an all-male setting can generate significant negative transference in the client as well as negative counter-transference in the clinician.[7]

Bob has a counselor assigned to him by an addiction treatment program. The counselor is divorced and harbors her own anger toward male clients who remind her of her abusive ex-husband. Bob is the current recipient of her negative counter-transference. Unfortunately, Bob experiences negative transference toward the counselor, too, as he sees her as a replica of his wife, who had been verbally abusive throughout their twenty-year marriage. The likelihood of developing a healthy therapeutic alliance is minimal without good supervision for Bob's counselor. It is more likely that he will not get his needs met.

Men as Clinicians in All-Male Settings
Men tend to address tasks more readily with male counselors. This predisposition may work more effectively in a treatment setting that utilizes brief, task-oriented therapy models involving solution-focused and Motivational Interviewing techniques. Men view their male counselors as more legitimate than their female counselors, thus giving the male clinician a greater sense of empowerment. Men seem to understand other men more easily than women do. In addition, men will disclose

some information to male counselors more readily than they will to female counselors.[8]

At the same time, there are problems that can ensue from employing men as clinicians in all-male settings. Some male clinicians may reinforce negative male communication patterns, such as referring to women in derogatory terms. Men from racial and cultural groups that have been traditionally disempowered by society may find it difficult to conceive of letting go of their power in keeping with the twelve-step concept of powerlessness. Perceiving themselves as having little power in society, they feel a need to retain whatever limited power they think they have. An example of this is the homeless man who has used his survival skills as his only form of power. To be asked to give up this power to survive may be more difficult for the man to hear from a male than a female counselor.

Gay men may experience or fear more heterosexism in an all-male setting. Likewise, in an all-male setting (especially one not sensitive to the traditional male values of competition and dominance) some men may be more preoccupied with the racial, ethnic, and cultural issues that separate them from other men and be less able to receive the benefits of looking at the things that participants share. Treatment staff, male or female, need to understand whatever biases men may bring to treatment.

Two: Overcoming Barriers for Men

Achieving coordinated treatment services for men is not an easy task, given the significant number of barriers to be overcome. In addition to the resistance and hesitancy of men to seek treatment in the first place, a number of environmental factors hinder the provision of appropriate care, such as:

- Uncoordinated treatment services

- Gaps in the availability of services

- A lack of research, and therefore understanding, about male-specific needs for care

- The disproportionate presence of women care providers

There is a need for better integration of treatment systems with other healthcare and related systems, such as the criminal justice system, workplace systems (Employee Assistance Programs, Human Resource Management Programs), faith-based systems, government-sponsored systems (Military Health Care Delivery, Welfare-to-Work, and family counseling), and community-based services and groups for men.

There is a lack of integration between residential/inpatient addiction services with outpatient services. The weakest link in most inpatient treatment programs is the lack of coordinated, continuing aftercare programs. Most men are released from residential care with simply a referral to a twelve-step program and a copy of that fellowship's basic text, and perhaps a referral to an outpatient therapist for counseling. Yet experience indicates that a minimum of six months of aftercare is needed to maximize the gains of residential treatment.

Some impediments to adequate, integrated substance-abuse treatment include shifts in funding for services, changes in legislative and other public policy priorities, and community attitudes about addiction, recovery, and men's issues. For example, a community may be far more receptive to offering services for women in recovery than for men, with a strong social stigma and prejudice against the male substance abuser. Community fears about potential violence and inappropriate sexual and other antisocial behavior also impede treatment.

Mental health problems of substance abusing clients are exacerbated by the failure of many systems to diagnose and/or treat co-occurring disorders (see previous discussion about men and depression), related healthcare concerns, aging and substance-abuse issues, and behavioral addictions (such as sex, gambling, and eating disorders).

There are difficulties in navigating the healthcare and social service systems. These systems are complicated, with time-consuming requirements of time documentation, as well as internal bickering about who is responsible for what services and which services take priority. Lack of education, chronic or acute medical or psychiatric complications, sexual disorders, developmental delays, and age-related difficulties are additional challenges to gaining access to the services.

The obstacles men face when they contemplate seeking care include:

- The cost of care, which is not always covered by insurance even if one has a policy

- Male-based shame, stigma, and discrimination[9]

- A sense of physical inadequacy

- Emotional inexpressiveness

- Difficulty with submitting to direction from female care providers

- A sense of intellectual inferiority or failure in meeting masculine standards of work

- A sense of sexual inadequacy, of not being enough of a "man" in bed, not able to adequately satisfy his partner

Stigma is often associated with cultural differences and sexual orientation, including societal homophobia and cultural biases against men seeking help.

Legal problems can be associated with recovery, including probation, incarceration, deportation, loss of child custody, lack of partner support, lack of support from family and friends, lack of transportation, language barriers, and other cultural issues.

Men who seek financial gain in an environment that lacks economic opportunity may be attracted to and become involved in criminal activity. There may be a lack of economic opportunities available for men who have been involved in criminal activities, such as illegal gambling, prostitution, drug running, or violent crime, setting the stage for a "Catch 22" situation where a man can't get off of the criminal treadmill.

The recovering man needs assistance in navigating treatment systems, particularly if the man lacks information or education on how to do so. The following factors have been found to affect retention of men in treatment: severity of addiction, involvement with the criminal justice system, employment issues, income, parenting responsibilities, and the therapeutic alliance.

Issues concerning men mandated to treatment also need to be addressed. Treatment practitioners should consider the following recommendations when designing programs for legally coerced clients:

- The period of intervention should be lengthy.

- Treatment programs should provide a high level of structure, particularly during the early stages of recovery.

- Programs must be flexible enough to meet the specific, unique needs of each male patient.

- Programs must undergo regular evaluation to determine their level of effectiveness and to detect changes in the client populations served.

- Vocational training should be provided as an adjunct to care, especially for mandated clients with limited skills and employability.

- A careful review of readiness and willingness to engage should be part of the program.

- Development and consistent implementation of protocols for disclosure of information, especially sensitive information that might affect the patient's future recovery, employability, return to society, and parental and familial roles.

Agencies can show their commitment to men by displaying positive images of men in brochures, waiting-room magazines, on occasions such as Father's Day, and in posters and artwork that depict men in a positive manner. Agency staff can "put out the welcome mat" for men, engaging men in informal, positive conversation, and showing them empathy in a variety of situations.

In addition, it is important for agencies to make a commitment to male involvement by advertising their desire for men as volunteers and participants in the agency's program literature, mission statement, and so forth. Agencies can find out what men want by asking what they are feeling or thinking at the time of their admission and how they feel they can be helpful to themselves and others as they go through the program.

Clinical staff should notice what men are doing and how they spend their time to see if they have sufficient activities in the moments when they are not in therapeutic sessions. It can be helpful to take a survey to find out what men might want from the program and what is not currently being offered that they would like to see become part of the program. Ask them. They will tell you.

Supervisors can conduct an environmental audit of their program to determine how to implement services for men. This can be done by bringing in a panel of men to discuss men's issues and concerns with staff.

It is important for agencies to address staff attitudes, including resistance about dealing with men, which negatively affect men's treatment. They can conduct training and discussions with staff, using the following kinds of statements and questions: "We do not have many men involved in our program. Why not?" and "We could involve more men if . . ."

Agencies can address resistance to men on the part of female staff. Male- or female-bashing among staff should not be condoned, of course, and appropriate boundaries need to be established.

Agencies can incorporate more men into the program by seeking out and hiring male staff and recruiting male volunteers. It is important for men to be incorporated into all aspects of the program, not just those geared to men's issues. Men will feel more comfortable in a setting where they see other men working and participating in activities.

It is also necessary for counselors to understand characteristics of male group behavior. Training and clinical supervision can be effectively utilized to increase clinicians' awareness of the patterns of "the things men do."

Three: Counseling Men: Structuring the Environment

There are a number of critical considerations in working with men. In a treatment model that includes both genders, decision-making about policy and procedures is improved when both gender's perspectives are considered. Mechanisms can be designed to receive input from the treatment providers and the receivers, to address issues of gender, race, culture, and sexual orientation, both among the providers, receivers of treatment, and between providers and receivers. Teamwork, cofacilitation of counseling, and collaborative working relationships between male and female staff benefit both the clinical team and the clients by providing positive role models for communication and cooperation between the genders. Agencies that treat primarily men will want to take into account the following critical considerations when designing or adapting their treatment programs for men.

Men who are antagonistic toward women in power may have difficulty forming a healthy therapeutic alliance with female counselors. Likewise, racial and sexual orientation issues are rarely brought up by either supervisors or clinicians in supervision.[10] The critical questions of sexual attraction between clients and clinicians, dual relationships, and boundary violations are also often raised in gender-specific groups, especially when there is a counselor of one gender treating a client of another. However, it is important to realize that sexual attraction and the risk of serious boundary violations occur in any gender configuration in clinical work. A number of sources provide useful guidance for clinicians and agencies concerning the wide range of ethical boundary dilemmas that arise in practice.[11]

Rather than scapegoat or blame the patient or clinician for these problems, the agency that has considered these issues and prepared for their discussion can bring them to that forum to discuss and resolve.

Likewise, it is essential that supervisors feel comfortable initiating the discussion of these issues with the clinician. It is the responsibility of both the clinician and the supervisor to discuss sensitive issues that affect the quality of services offered to the client.

Structuring All-Male Treatment Groups

The structure of an all-male group is important. Men learn the rules of the game early, in the playground, on the ball field, or in other sports and competitive arenas. Therefore, group norms and rules are critical for men. The explicit expectation is that all members (including the staff members) be in place at group and ready to go when the group is scheduled to begin. Groups can benefit from some degree of structure, beginning with a check-in period and an arriving and gathering ritual, in which each man takes an uninterrupted turn to describe his week/

day and to report on commitments made previously. A "jump ball" time is the period in which men begin the work of the group. Sessions can end with closing statements, an ending ritual in which each member has a brief period to summarize his experiences of the session and to offer a behavioral commitment—something he will work on.

Confidentiality—knowing that what is said stays within the walls of the group meeting room—is very important for the safety of any group and can be supported by a specific group rule about it. It is essential, especially when working with men, to negotiate the limits of confidentiality within the boundaries of the duty to warn/protect. Counselors utilize standard techniques when negotiating these boundaries. In addition, group comfort standards are required, as well as a model of accountability wherein each man is expected to make and keep his promises. There are also opportunities for humor and lighthearted emotional outbursts, homework assignments, coaching, and "instant replay and slow motion" periods in which the counselor can stop the action for a process check. Other group procedures include role playing behaviors, show-and-tell times when men can demonstrate their responses and actions, and therapist modeling and self-disclosure periods. Confrontations need to be customized to the needs and issues of each man, and positive behavior needs to be recognized and acknowledged. Male mentorship among the group members is also important, as men are mimetic, that is, they have a tendency to model themselves after and to follow other men.

Screening and Assessment

When treatment professionals consider issues of screening and assessment of men with chemical dependency problems, they must be aware of the ways in which male gender, discussed in previous sections, influences the help-seeking behavior of men.

What can be done to engage a man in the screening and assessment process?

Often, men are ambivalent about seeking help for behavioral health problems, so it is useful for the clinician to understand, as much as possible, what set of circumstances prompted a man's help-seeking behavior. Perhaps the most important questions a counselor can ask a male client are "Why are you here?" "Why now?" "What problem do you need help with?" and "How can I help you?"

Understanding the phases of motivation for change, ambivalence, and action illuminates all forms of treatment and is especially helpful when addressing male issues in treatment. Given that most men are brought up in a way that discourages seeking help for personal issues, clinicians working with chemically dependent men should expect to find ambivalence toward change along with possible fear, which may look like resistance, in the face of external pressure or coercion.

When beginning the screening process, the counselor can conceptualize the engagement process as a series of steps in which the male client can move from stage to stage, from screening to treatment to continuing care. Men are goal-oriented, so breaking the process down into smaller goals is helpful to engage men in their treatment from the outset. The primary goal of each clinical contact should be to engage the man in a conversation about his life that encourages him to return for the next visit. So, take it one step at a time. That is, even if treatment is clearly indicated, the counselor may first want to elicit agreement to do an initial screening to determine whether further assessment, followed by treatment, is warranted and acceptable to the client.

Emphasizing the immediate goal of each step, from screening to assessment to treatment to continuing care, can be reassuring to a man who is goal-oriented. The counselor can present each stage of treatment with a clear plan for what will happen and what the next steps might be.

Measurable results will be part of this plan and contract. A letter documenting the visit, attendance, or phone call can provide tangible evidence of movement for the man. Giving the man something to do, a specific task, to prepare for the next session can facilitate engagement and support his sense of confidence, control, and efficacy. It also supports the collaborative nature of treatment, emphasizing the client's freedom of choice.

Similarly, the counselor may wish to acknowledge explicitly the difficulty men have seeking assistance. If the client expresses the concern that his need for treatment is a sign of failure or weakness, reframe such comments by defining help-seeking behavior as a sign of strength and courage. Paying attention to the level of emotional intensity, particularly early in the process, and being respectful of the man's expression of emotion, creates a safe environment for the man and the counselor to work together. Allowing the man to set his level of emotional exploration assures a mutual working alliance.

Clinicians who stay aware of the interpersonal intensity of initial interactions will be able to weather the variations within the therapeutic alliance in a way that permits greatest advancement for the client. Again, avoiding competitive exchanges, comments, or questions that might provoke shame builds the therapeutic alliance. To decrease the potentially uncomfortable intensity of close contact with a counselor (especially if the counselor is a woman), it may help to sit with the man at an angle or side-by-side rather than directly face-to-face. During clinical assessment, men may prefer more physical distance between the clinician and the client. In some settings, talking while walking and other strategies that decrease the intensity of direct eye contact may help the man feel more comfortable.

Eco-maps, genograms and family maps (diagrams of one's family of origin), timelines of one's life, and graphs of scores on screening and assessment measures can be used to create the kind of concrete, visual representations with which some men are more comfortable working.[12]

For further information on conducting a comprehensive assessment of substance-abusing men, we refer you to TIP 24, "A Guide to Substance Abuse Services for Primary Care Physicians."[13]

In summary, there are three steps in a comprehensive substance-abuse assessment:

1. The screening phase (previously discussed),

2. The problem assessment phase, and

3. The personal assessment phase.

Gender-sensitive problem assessment includes consideration of psychosocial adaptation, substance use patterns, and help-seeking behavior of men. The assessment also can also be sensitive to ways in which age, ethnicity, socioeconomic status, geographic location, and sexual orientation contribute to differences in values, attitudes, and behavioral dispositions to substance use and abuse. That is, while considering ways men are alike because of their gender, clinicians must also be sensitive to ways in which men differ from one another.

Retrospective methods (looking back on one's life) using timelines and follow-back procedures define the nature and consequences of substance use during a specified period of time. Again, because men tend to be more comfortable analyzing data, visual presentation of substance use and consequences of use along a timeline or on a calendar may be a more gender-sensitive manner to collect and display the information to a male client.

Future-oriented or prospective methods using calendars or other means of personal record-keeping can document patterns and consequences of use. Laboratory studies are also used in screening to document recent use, obtain markers of chronic use, and document medical consequences of chronic use.

Standardized assessment approaches are available for both the problem assessment and the personal assessment.

For the personal assessment phase of the comprehensive assessment, standardized instruments such as the Addiction Severity Index[14] are often used for historical and concurrent problem assessment. It is important to distinguish between confirmatory and compensatory drinking and drug use for men. Confirmatory styles of use involve using alcohol and other drugs because it is consistent with personal definitions of masculinity that men have integrated into their definitions of self. Compensatory styles of use involve using alcohol and other drugs to shore up a tenuous sense of one's self as a man or to deal with stress associated with perceived failure to meet traditional male gender role expectations.[15] Other male-sensitive instruments are the Male Role Norm Scale,[16] the Gender Role Conflict Scale,[17] and the Masculine Gender Role Stress Scale.[18] Other, more in-depth instruments that are male-sensitive are the Brannon Masculinity Scale[19] and the Male Role Norms Inventory.[20]

Because there are clear links between poor physical health and chronic substance abuse in men, any comprehensive substance abuse assessment must include a complete physical examination. Ideally, the exam will include lab studies to screen both for health problems associated with the use of specific drugs and for health problems more generally associated with men. If the male client is being seen in a hospital or residential setting, a complete physical exam with lab studies should always be part of the routine admission process. In ambulatory settings, the initial interview should include questions about health history, general nutrition, sleep patterns, weight changes, last physical examination, and last dental examination. In addition, when feasible, a full personality assessment is beneficial, including the following areas:

- Antisocial personality and mental health status
- Motivational levels
- Family history
- Childhood and other trauma
- Criminality, anger, and physical violence history
- Sexual functioning
- Risk-taking behavior
- Personal relationships
- Educational history, vocational background, and leisure activities
- Spirituality/religious background and orientation

As some of the more sensitive issues arise, shame will often be present. It might be helpful for the clinician to explore that shame through reflections and questions such as "You feel ashamed about _____. Can you describe what that's like? How often do you sense that, feel that way?" Responses to these short questions can be used to quantify the frequency and intensity of reactions such as shame, guilt, and anxiety. The Internalized Shame Scale[21] is an exceptional tool for assessment of male clients.

Four: Clinical Approaches to Treating Men

The clinician's role is to assist male clients in developing communication skills; in differentiating among being assertive, passive, and aggressive; and in learning how to say no (refusal skills) or to take "no" for an answer. The counselor can talk about and model how to treat women with respect and give women power to consent without intimidation. Some male clients may benefit from learning listening and conflict resolution skills, especially to begin with the words "I feel . . ." or "I am . . ." when expressing an emotion.

Offering nonviolent role models to male clients, as well as encouraging empathy and talking about feelings are two ways that counselors can help men expand their emotional experience and vocabulary. Counselors can teach men fathering skills, including affirming, caring, nurturing, forgiving, patience, and vulnerability. Opportunities to engage in activities that encourage reflection, expression of emotion, and nurturing—such as art, poetry, music, and community service—are welcome alternatives to more traditional male activities. Clinicians can support nonviolent sports that foster cooperation, bonding, and commitment, while affirming new, less physical, less competitive activities (e.g., canoeing, solving puzzles, hiking) as alternatives to the traditional male preoccupation with competition and violent sports. Clients can benefit from a forum in which they can discuss how violence (sexual or other) has affected them and other men, and explore what part they can play in the solution to violence in our culture.

Case History: Joe

Joe has a history of violence at home, physically abusing his wife and children. He has difficulty with anger management and impulse control.

For years Joe has been in and out of jails and addiction treatment programs that never addressed his anger. Each time, upon discharge, he'd return to the same pattern, using alcohol as a tool so that he could vent his anger. Finally, Joe finds a treatment program that addresses his anger. As part of this treatment for his addiction the counselors teach Joe how to control his temper, how to find other, nonviolent forms of release, and how to communicate calmly with his family.

After a year of group counseling, Joe is in recovery and his family life is significantly improved.

In an age of heightened awareness of cultural, racial, sexual orientation, and gender issues, it is important for clinicians working with substance-abusing men to know the concerns of specific subpopulations and cultures. Economic circumstances and their related social and psychological problems introduce a common set of challenges and tend to create a lower quality of life for many people, especially people of color.[22] Low socioeconomic status is the most prominent common factor in the lives of many African-Americans, Hispanics, Asian-Americans, and American Indians. Low levels of education, underemployment, and lack of health insurance, resulting in limited access to healthcare and consequent exacerbation of health problems, are generally associated with lower socioeconomic status and higher substance abuse rates. Understanding and addressing the impact of these cultural characteristics can help agencies and clinicians respond more fully and accurately to their male clients' needs.

A good first step in treating men is to acknowledge cultural issues and develop greater cultural competency with men.

Bell and others have written extensively about substance abuse and ethnicity. Further study is needed with respect to substance abuse and sexual orientation (including bisexuality), substance abuse and older men, geographic subcultures (such as rural vs. urban lifestyles for men as well as inner-city behavior), and substance abuse in the context of physical disabilities.

Further, drug-specific treatment components are necessary to address the full range of behaviors of substance-abusing men. Finally, relapse-prevention strategies specific to men need to be designed.

Motivational Enhancement

Motivation is considered a major component of personal change and growth. Motivation is multifaceted and constantly fluctuating along many dimensions. Healthcare providers note that men can be difficult to get into treatment for any health-related problem, especially substance abuse, and that motivation for care is a critical factor in involving men in treatment. Men seem to require different levels of motivational engagement that depend not only on the substances used and their consequences, but also on the degree to which men believe in and support values that are consistent with their traditional concepts of what it means to behave like a man.

These values and perceptions are not fixed, but do in fact constantly change to some extent as men go through life. One obvious challenge is to help men find their own motivation to overcome some of these commonly accepted male attitudes that deter them from seeking help for their substance-abuse problems. One way to enhance this motivation is to change the structure and strategies of the treatment program to be more responsive to the habits and psychosocial needs of the men served. We previously discussed some recommendations about how to adapt your programs along these lines.

Men often complain they feel as if they are treated like children by care providers as well as educators. This decreases their motivation to follow through with treatment, especially in inpatient settings. Men's socialization around power seeking, control, and self-reliance works against some current treatment modalities. Perhaps the greatest challenge for substance-abuse treatment providers has more to do with changing our societal views and assumptions about men and manhood than with treatment itself. Tailoring treatment specifically for men has to start before a man comes to a healthcare provider if we want to change the current trend that a man is more likely never to come to treatment than he is to present himself voluntarily.

We highly recommend the utilization of Motivational Interviewing (MI) as a means to create relationship and help each man find his own intrinsic motivation. Skilled use of MI can have a positive effect on behavioral change.[23]

External circumstances (for example, a failed marriage, a court order, loss of a job, or an EAP referral) may force a man to seek help before he elects to do so on his own initiative. Media attention to male attitudes about healthcare and help-seeking can also provide some form of external impetus to change men's healthcare behavior. Changing how men are socialized, however, will probably yield more positive results than any changes we bring to treatment programs. Encouraging more positive attitudes regarding emotional expression and help-seeking behavior in men can bring about a change from self-perceived weakness to one of strength and courage of full expression.

Twelve-Step Programs

The issues particularly relevant for men in recovery that twelve-step programs typically address include the following: a sense of isolation and loneliness; power and powerlessness; trauma and crisis; judgment, comparing, contrasting, and competing; sponsorship and mentoring with other men; and spirituality. These are areas in which twelve-step programs are particularly helpful for men, providing a safe and accepting environment where men can address these issues. Closed meetings for men are useful in opening men up to such issues in ways they might not otherwise feel safe or comfortable doing.

Therefore, we highly recommend a program of twelve-step recovery as a component of men's treatment when chemical dependency or another behavioral/process dependency (sex, gambling, food) is present. Such programs provide an environment and meeting place that is rarely found or available to men except in faith communities. Just think about it: where else do men gather except in bars or sporting events, all of which center around drinking, drugging, or competition?

Outpatient vs. Residential Services

For some men, such as the homeless or men suffering from late-stage addiction and co-occurring disorders, special considerations are needed with respect to the location and type of treatment. Housing status, employment capabilities, detoxification and medical status, and potential recovery resources are all things to consider when the counselor and the man are determining the best fit for services. The American Society of Addiction Medicine (ASAM) Patient Placement Criteria (PPC-2) is most helpful in finding the right placement level for patients. As men have higher rates of criminal behavior, homelessness, and medical complications than women, these considerations need to be factored in when finding or making the proper patient placement.

Numerous studies have been done on the efficacy of outpatient versus inpatient treatment.[24] However, there is a paucity of studies on patient placement when applied to the treatment needs of men specifically. Although residential treatment had been the modality of choice for quite some time, reductions in funding have devalued the status of residential care ("twenty-eight-day treatment") as the gold standard for rehabilitation. However, in light of newly recognized male-specific concerns, researchers may need to revisit the efficacy of outpatient services for particular men dealing with such issues.

Other potential components to be considered in designing a continuum of services for men are shelters, transitional living arrangements, half- and quarter-way housing, emergency seasonal housing/shelters, and domiciliary arrangements.

Individual Counseling

The National Institute of Drug Abuse (NIDA) Individual Drug Counseling Model outlines strategies for counseling on a one-on-one basis.[25] The key questions are, "Who is most likely to benefit from individual counseling?" and "When is it the most beneficial?" It may be easier for some men to engage in individual counseling because they do not have to deal with their image and interpersonal issues in front of a group of people. For such a man, it will be much easier to discuss sensitive issues and deal with emotions and tears in privacy with a trained professional than it would be with a group of peers whom he will face again after admitting to or revealing aspects of himself that he normally would not share with other men. Although the group is bound to confidentiality, a professional enjoys a different level of trust from the client's perspective, especially given legal and ethical constraints. Also, the counselor is not seen as a peer or potential friend, but rather as someone providing a service in a context-specific relationship that is very personal, but very circumscribed in time, setting, and purpose.

Family Intervention

Family work has a long history in the substance abuse treatment field. However, family-oriented interventions pursued with men must be sensitive to the effects of gender role socialization on the client and his family life. The following areas need to be addressed:

- The influence of gender role socialization on the presenting problem
- Shared responsibility for change in the relationship
- Actively challenging stereotypical attitudes and behaviors
- Family-oriented engagement: promoting self-care for family

members, decreasing the risks of domestic violence, promoting communication between the substance-abusing individual and his partner, and reinforcing the client's and family's efforts to function on a daily basis

- Marital intervention to promote an atmosphere of abstinence, mutual respect, and open and healthy communication between partners

- Parenting intervention: fathering roles, childcare responsibilities, the male partner's responsibility for sexual reproduction, problematic attitudes about parenting, socially responsible parenting, healing father-child breaches, overcoming longstanding generational parenting issues (including family-of-origin issues), legal barriers to effective parenting, improving the relationship with mothers (who typically control access to children), improving communication skills with children, specific parenting skills, overcoming family secrets about substance abuse and related behaviors, and aiding the substance-abusing father in providing emotional support to children

- Addressing violence issues, including domestic violence or child abuse and neglect perpetrated against or by the addict

- Legal assistance with family court matters, including divorce, child custody, child support, allegations of abuse or neglect, child welfare and family court systems, and societal stereotypes of substance-abusing men as indifferent, uninvolved, irresponsible, and irrelevant

- Reproductive responsibility, unplanned paternity, intimacy disorders, communication patterns, gender stereotyping, sexual misconceptions, social pressures associated with sex roles and gender, sexual health, risky sexual behaviors, and pregnancy-related questions

Counseling Strategies

It is important to be aware of the male socialization process and the conditioning that goes with it. Having a vision of the person underneath the conditioning (his innate characteristics and capacities) and offering it to the male client is central to a sense of hope and a strong therapeutic alliance. For example, it is essential that the care providers show that they know the man is good, caring, likable, or capable—even if his actions or the way he displays his distress does not show you these qualities in the moment.

The way men display their conditioning is a road map to the hurt they have endured. The distress-laden ways in which men at times act, for instance, often reflect either how they were treated or how they learned to act, to cope with the way they were treated. In this way, the counselor can separate the man from his conditioning and focus on the former, while acknowledging the latter.

Because of narrowly defined expectations and their inability to recover from hurt, men often lose track of very basic needs. These needs get channeled in other, often inappropriate ways. The counselor can look for the real underlying needs. For example, often men's longing for sex is really a longing for caring, with no other accepted avenue to feel it. Men's violence is often an expression of feeling out of control and uncontained. Their real need is for structure and for experiencing control of their internal environment.

It is helpful for the care provider to learn to help men face the feelings that lie beneath their attachments to people, objects, sensations, and experiences. Some examples might include:

- Women: affection, softness, other "feminine qualities"
- Children: play, pride, ownership

- Cars: freedom, control

- Work: self-worth

- Competition: self-worth, a place in the world

- Alcohol: relief, freedom from stress (of course, addiction will take on a control of its own)

Men's attachments to their coping styles are as deep as they needed to be to survive persistent attacks they had to cope with during the conditioning process. Men will cling to those strategies until it is clearly safe to let go. Thus, the counselor should not attack men for these struggles, nor expect them to readily accept his or her attempts to assist them in exploring their conditioning. Instead, it is important to hold men accountable for their effect on others and offer a hand toward making a change in behavior when they recognize a need to do so.

In offering a man a way out of conditioned styles of coping, a care provider will often uncover and encounter the feelings (anger, rage, loneliness, desperation) that were swallowed when he initially succumbed to the conditioning. Expect and welcome these feelings and help the man process them and behave appropriately.

Many men show sensitivity to feelings, but have major barriers to releasing them; counselors can help with both.

Counselors can use positive, socially accepted male language to encourage and support men as they look at themselves. "It's brave of you to share your feelings." "It will be helpful to others, too, if you face these issues." "There is much more ahead for you if we look at this."

The male training is to be decisive, opinionated. It is important to honor the other ways men have been able to cope with situations or manage and help men live with ambiguity.

Counseling with a man has a tremendous potential power due to the intimacy that may be experienced by the male client. Most men have not been offered much closeness in their lives. A counseling experience may give a man a remarkably higher quality of one-to-one attention than he has ever experienced. Respect this, pace things well, and enjoy and use this opportunity to help him move forward.

The safe environment that the counselor creates to build and maintain the therapeutic alliance permits the expression of sexual feelings without shame. Most men have had feelings of shame heaped on their sexual feelings and consequently remain secretive in these areas.

If it is safe for you, allow the possibility that the client may experience sexual feelings for you as a male or female therapist. There are specific techniques that can help work on these feelings, but acknowledging them may be a good start. If the counselor is male, issues around sexual orientation, including homophobia, may arise, creating an opportunity for the client to explore his relationship with his sexual orientation. Perhaps, above all, if a counselor can offer a man a bridge to the neglected parts of himself, he may receive a tremendous antidote to his socialization.

Section III Notes

1. Sharon S. Brehm, *Intimate Relationships* (New York: Random House, 1985).

2. Irvin D. Yalom, *Theory and Practice of Group Psychotherapy* (New York: Basic Books, 1970).

3. Warren Farrell, *Why Men Are the Way They Are: The Male-Female Dynamic* (Columbus: McGraw-Hill, 1986) pp. 139–40.

4. Deborah Tannen, *You Just Don't Understand: Women and Men in Conversation* (New York: William Morrow, 1990) pp. 76–7.

5. Gwen Webber, "Feminist Models of Supervision," presented at American Association for Marriage and Family Therapy (AAMFT) Annual Conference, 1991.

6. Carol Gilligan, *In a Different Voice: Psychological Theory and Women's Development* (Cambridge: Harvard University Press, 1992).

7. Charlene Alderfer, "The Effects of Gender on the Supervisory Process" (EdD diss., University of Massachusetts, 1991).

8. Ibid.

9. Paul W. Efthim et al., "Gender role stress in relation to shame, guilt, and externalization," *Journal of Counseling and Development*, volume 79, number 4 (2001): pp. 430–38.

10. Webber, "Feminist Models of Supervision." Alderfer, "The Effects of Gender on the Supervisory Process."

11. Jerry Edelwich and Archie Brodsky, Sexual Dilemmas for the Helping Professional: Revised and Expanded Edition (New York: Routledge, 1991). Richard S. Epstein, *Keeping Boundaries: Maintaining Safety and Integrity in the Psychotherapeutic Process* (Washington, DC: American Psychiatric Press, 1994). Thomas G. Gutheil and Archie Brodsky, *Preventing Boundary Violations in Clinical Practice* (New York: Guilford Press, 2008). Frederic G. Reamer, *Tangled Relationships: Managing Boundary Issues in the Human Services* (New York: Columbia University Press, 2001).

12. Diane F. Halpern, "The disappearance of cognitive gender differences: What you see depends on where you look," *American Psychologist*, volume 44, number 8 (1989): pp. 1156–58.

13. Center for Substance Abuse Treatment, "A Guide to Substance Abuse Services for Primary Care Clinicians" (Rockville: Substance Abuse and Mental Health Services Administration, 1997). (Treatment Improvement Protocol (TIP) Series, No. 24. Available from http://www.ncbi.nlm.nih.gov/books/NBK64827.)

14. Robert Mathias, "The Addiction Severity Index," *NIDA Notes*, volume 9, number 2 (1994): pp. 8–9.

15. Robert J. Williams and Lina A. Ricciardelli, "Gender congruence in confirmatory and compensatory drinking," *The Journal of Psychology*, volume 133, issue 3 (1999): pp. 323–31.

16. Edward H. Thompson, Jr. and Joseph H. Pleck, "The structure of male role norms," *American Behavioral Scientist*, volume 29 (1986): 531–43.

17. James M. O'Neil et al., "Fifteen years of theory and research on men's gender role conflict: New paradigms for empirical research," in *A New Psychology of Men*, Eds. Ronald F. Levant and William S. Pollack (New York: Basic Books, 1995).

18. Richard M. Eisler, "The relationship between masculine gender role stress and men's health risk: The validation of a construct," in *A New Psychology of Men*, Eds. Ronald F. Levant and William S. Pollack (New York: Basic Books, 1995): pp. 207–25

19. Robert Brannon and Samuel Juni, "A scale for measuring attitudes about masculinity," *Psychological Documents*, volume 14, number 1 (1984).

20. Ronald F. Levant et al., "The male role: An investigation of contemporary norms," *Journal of Mental Health Counseling*, volume 14, issue 3 (1992): pp. 325–37.

21. David R. Cook, "Internalized shame scale," (Menomonie: University of Wisconsin-Stout, 1989).

22. Katrina W. Johnson et al., "Panel II: Macrosocial and environmental influences on minority health," *Health Psychology*, volume 14, number 7 (1995): pp. 601–12.

23. William Miller and Stephen Rollnick, *Motivational Interviewing: Preparing People for Change* (New York: Guilford Press, 2002).

24. William R. Miller and Reid K. Hester, "Treating the problem drinker: Modern approaches," in *The Addictive Behaviors: Treatment of Alcoholism, Drug Abuse, Smoking, and Obesity*, Ed. William R. Miller (Oxford: Pergamon Press, 1980) 111–41. William R. Miller et al., "What works? A summary of alcohol treatment outcome research," in *Handbook of Alcoholism Treatment Approaches: Effective Alternatives*, Eds. Reid K. Hester and William R. Miller (Boston: Allyn and Bacon, 2003) pp. 13–63.

25. Delinda E. Mercer and George E. Woody, "An Individual Drug Counseling Approach to Treat Cocaine Addiction: The Collaborative Cocaine Treatment Study Model," National Institute on Drug Abuse (NIDA) Therapy Manuals for Drug Abuse, Manual 3. Available from http://archives.drugabuse.gov/TXManuals/IDCA/IDCA1.html.

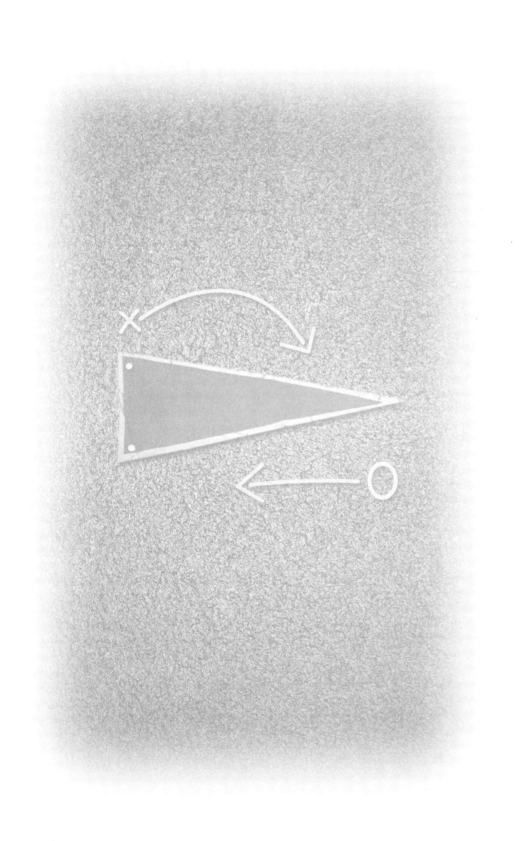

Section IV: Resources for Healing

One: Homework

What's the simplest way to make a good counseling session even better? Give the client a homework assignment. Just how powerful are homework assignments? One homework assignment literally altered the face of treatment.

In an interview shortly before his death, Albert Ellis, the father of Rational Emotive Behavior Therapy (REBT), told the interviewer a fascinating story about a landmark psychotherapeutic homework assignment he gave himself that spawned the REBT movement and changed the course of counseling and therapy for at least the next fifty years.

At age nineteen, Ellis was petrified at the thought of approaching women. Two hundred days a year he would go to the Bronx Botanical Garden in New York wanting to meet women but not having the courage to initiate conversation. Ellis began reading the work of the early behaviorists suggesting that if you confronted your fears they would often disappear. So, in the words of Albert Ellis, "I gave myself a famous homework assignment in August."* Each day he challenged himself to approach every single woman who was alone on a park bench and talk to her. "I'll give myself one minute, one lousy minute," he told himself, "and if I die . . . well . . . I die." He approached more than one hundred women. Thirty immediately got up and walked away (not too bad considering Ellis did his homework assignment in New York City, not known for its friendliness to strangers). Out of all the women only one made a date with him, and she subsequently didn't show up. The good news was that Ellis overcame his fear of approaching women.

From that point on, homework became one of the bedrocks of his theory.

What type of therapist uses homework assignments? A better question might be, what type of therapist doesn't? In fact, psychotherapeutic homework is used by individual therapists, group therapists, and marriage and family counselors. In addition to rational emotive therapy and reality therapy, counselors practicing assertiveness training, behavior therapy, cognitive behavior therapy, conditioned reflex therapy, gestalt therapy, career counseling, neurolinguistic programming, transactional analysis, person-centered therapy, brief-strategic or solution-oriented therapy, and logotherapy, to name a few, use homework assignments in their counseling practices.

Homework assignments take advantage of the fact that most people are adept at modeling the behavior of others, as well as anticipating what others will say or do. The use of homework allows patients to progress at a faster rate and flourish as if they were receiving additional sessions (something we can all use in the age of managed care). Another

---

* Used with the permission of the Albert Ellis Institute.

plus when working with a substance-abusing client is that homework assignments zero in on one of a substance abuser's worst hurdles: what to do when an uncontrollable urge to engage in an addictive behavior occurs outside the treatment setting.

Homework assignments may not be appropriate for the first session or two. Literature has shown that the counselor should meet with the client a minimum of three or four sessions before prescribing homework assignments.[1] We do not necessarily agree with this assessment, for we have had good success—with men in particular—using homework assignments early in the therapeutic relationship.

Also, the counselor can tailor the assignment to the client's specific addictive behavior. One way to introduce the exercise to the client is to say, "I have noticed that you are an extremely perceptive person. For instance, you seem to know exactly what your boss is going to say. In the last session you suggested that your brother would call you and ask you to go drinking on Monday night, and he did. I have seen you for nine sessions now and you probably have an excellent idea of what I'm going to say and how I'm going to say it. So here's what I want you to do, if you are willing," (it is important here to get permission for the upcoming directive).

"Whenever you get the uncontrollable urge to drink (gamble, etc.), I want you to begin a dialogue as if you were right here in my office. In other words, based on what you have learned in our sessions, I want you to tell me about your urges and then play the part of me and respond to yourself. If you are not sure what I would say, just take an educated guess. You can write it in a journal or record the imaginary session into a tape recorder. Bring your journal or your tape to the next session so we can examine it."

In many cases the mere act of creating the make-believe session curbs the client's urge to engage in the addictive behavior. The beauty of this simple exercise is that it teaches the client to think like a counselor, which is one of the most important goals of treatment or rehabilitation.

Finally, counselors should challenge themselves to create their own innovative homework assignments. The following are recommendations to help the counselor develop his or her own materials and assignments:

- Use only assignments with which you feel comfortable.

- Carry out the strategy in a spirit of empathy and optimism.

- Always check ethical guidelines prior to implementing any technique.

- Use caution to ensure that clients are not embarrassed or physically harmed by the assignment.

- If you are new to the field or undergoing close supervision for licensure or certification, check with your clinical supervisor before you prescribe a homework assignment to be certain it fits within the therapeutic model of the agency at which you are working.

- Role play the homework assignment with a trained colleague or supervisor before attempting it for the first time with a client.

- Never attempt a technique for which you have no training or clinical supervision.

- Do not assume that even an effective homework assignment will work in every case.

- Do not assume that a homework assignment that worked well with a client will work effectively with the same client at a later date.

- Provide a clear rationale for the assignment, linked to the person's mutually agreed-on goals.

- Always take multicultural and diversity considerations into account.

- Use only language the client can understand. Be as specific as possible.

- "Bend, fold, and mutilate" existing strategies to increase your comfort level and to meet the needs of the client.

- Realize that some homework assignments need to be used repeatedly to be effective.

- Realize that therapeutic timing can make or break a technique.

Two: Bibliotherapy and Videotherapy

Most people realize how therapeutic reading a book or watching a film or DVD can be. When we read we enter the world described in the pages of a book and become involved with the characters in the story. When we read a good book or see a good film, we often leave the experience having gained new insight and ideas.

This is the purpose of bibliotherapy and/or videotherapy: to assist a client in overcoming the emotional turmoil related to a real-life problem by having him read literature or see a film on that topic. The story can then serve as a springboard for discussion in counseling and possible resolution of the dilemma. The care provider can offer guidance in the resolution of personal issues through the use of directed readings and follow-up activities.

The client is appropriate for bibliotherapy and/or videotherapy after he goes through three stages or tests:

1. **Identification:** the client is able to identify with a book or film character and events in the story, either real or fictitious. Sometimes it is best to have a character of approximately the client's age facing similar events.

2. **Catharsis:** the client is able to become emotionally involved in the story and can work to release pent-up emotions in counseling.

3. **Insight:** the client, after catharsis (with the help of the counselor), can become aware that his problems might also be addressed or solved. He can identify possible solutions to the character's and his own personal problems.

This work can be done in individual, family, or group therapy. In individual bibliotherapy or videotherapy, the material is assigned to a client for a specific need. The client may read or watch the material independently or it may be presented to him. The activities that follow the presentation are also conducted individually with the client. After discussing the material with his therapist, the client may be asked to do homework by speaking his responses into a tape recorder, writing them down in a journal, or expressing them artistically. Through this process the client is able to unblock destructive emotions and relieve emotional pressures.

Additionally, by examination and analysis of moral values and the stimulation of critical thinking, the client can develop greater self-awareness, an enhanced self-concept, and improved personal and social judgment. This outcome should result in improved behavior, an ability to handle and understand important life issues, and increased empathy, tolerance, respect, and acceptance of others, all through identification with an appropriate literary model.

When bibliotherapy or videotherapy is used with groups, the patients read or watch together, or listen while the counselor reads to them. Group discussion and activities follow. Clients become aware that they are not alone in their feelings and that their perceived problems are shared by others.

When doing this kind of work with men, the therapist treats the characters as co-counselors, aiding in the therapeutic process and relationship. The purpose of bibliotherapy and video work is to augment, not replace, therapy. The goal of this work is not to analyze the material for its literary quality, but to gain personal insights.

The counselor may "test drive" a book or a film before recommending it to clients. This involves reading or viewing the material and thinking about how it addresses a problem from your past or present experience. It is helpful to test drive it by inviting a colleague, friend, or family member to read or view and discuss the material with you, noting the characters with whom all parties identify and what emotions and insights are demonstrated.

Although bibliotherapy and videotherapy encourage change within the individual, their use is not restricted to crisis situations. It is not a cure-all, however, for deeply rooted psychological problems. Some deep-seated issues may best be resolved through more intensive therapeutic interventions. For instance, some clients, not yet able to view themselves in a literary mirror, may use literature for escape only. Others may tend to rationalize their problems away rather than face them. Still others may not be able to transfer insights into real life. Nonetheless, guided vicarious experiences with literary characters may prove to be helpful for many patients.

Clinicians need to be critical and careful in the use of the types of material that is chosen. Because of visual media's unavoidable, graphic nature and realistic portrayal of life issues, not every man is a suitable candidate for video work. Men with serious psychopathology or severe symptoms are not candidates for film work; neither are young boys. Attention to violence, even so-called "mild" violence is suggested; it may act as a trigger for past or ongoing trauma.

Bibliotherapy

In an age when self-help books fill sections of bookstores, when individuals often search these shelves or the Internet for help with problems, bibliotherapy may have reached a new high in utility to clients. It has been used in clinical practice for decades. There are several valuable texts and research studies that discuss the use of homework and bibliotherapy in counseling. A reading we recommend for this section is Janice M. Joshua and Donna DiMenna's, *Read Two Books and Let's Talk Next Week*.

Among the many benefits to homework assignments and bibliotherapy:

- To help clinicians track clinical progress and modify treatment[2]
- To enable clients to practice what they have learned in therapy[3]
- To maximize the effects of therapy on the client's world[4]
- To lead to greater self-reliance[5]
- To serve as a bridge between the client's therapy and real life
- To increase the client's awareness of his issues
- To increase emotional regulation and catharsis, bringing feelings to light through the use of the printed page
- To increase interpersonal effectiveness by reading about individuals who have overcome adversity and resolved their issues

- To overcome obstacles by finding solutions in the lives and accomplishments of others

A bibliography is included in Appendix I.

Videotherapy

Today, men like to watch movies and do video work more than they like reading. Our culture seems to be more visual than ever, and men prefer the visual mode. Films are fun, require small amounts of time and money, fit into the average man's busy routine, and enable him to readily identify with dilemmas of those portrayed in film and to easily recall plots and characters. Video and film combine realism with imagination and act as a therapeutic metaphor, providing the male client with a visual portrayal of something he might be feeling or living with.

Visual media have many positive features. Many men like films. Therefore, recommending a film to a male client and having him view it is generally a pleasant part of treatment. Films also overcome language barriers since most DVDs today have subtitles in various languages and are accessible to those who are homebound and may not be able to go to a theater or may not have a social life due to their geographic confinement. DVDs viewed at home can provide an avenue to growth and learning. A vast number of titles can be downloaded straight to your TV. Movies and films can be shared with family and friends, allowing for dialogue and exchange, especially for men who might not be part of a counseling program or are unwilling to participate in therapy. Films enhance rapport-building and the deepening of the therapeutic alliance between the counselor and the client.

Movies often are in the client's vernacular, taking the discussion out of the psychobabble of the counseling room and putting it in the common language of most men; and films and the media raise a level of curiosity for most clients, encouraging change and growth through "benign" interventions.

Films aid in treatment planning in at least seven ways:

1. They offer hope and encouragement to clients, such as the release illustrated in the film *The Shawshank Redemption*.

2. They provide an opportunity to reframe the problem, as in *Starting Over*.

3. They provide positive male role models for success and significance, as in *Rudy*.

4. They offer a means of identifying and reinforcing the client's internal strengths, as portrayed in *Parenthood* and *A River Runs Through It*.

5. They dramatize emotions, as in *The Son's Room* and *This Boy's Life*.

6. They aid in improving communication between men and their partners or family members, as shown in *The Accidental Tourist*.

7. They aid in prioritizing values, meaning, and purpose, as in the challenging and troubling movie *Short Cuts*.

A videography is included in Appendix II.

How to Use Bibliotherapy and Videotherapy

Choosing Materials

1. Identify the client's needs. This task is done through observation, counseling sessions, and a review of the client's records.

2. Match the client with appropriate materials. Offer books and films that deal with the presenting issue: divorce, a death in the family, or whatever needs have been identified, keeping the following in mind:

- What is the client's reading/language level?

- What interests him?

- Are the characters believable enough that the client can identify with them?

- Is the plot realistic and does it involve creative problem-solving?

3. Familiarize yourself with the material (read or see and understand it) before using it.

4. Decide on the setting and time for the biblio- or videotherapy assignment and how the patient will be introduced to the material.

Using the Materials

Review these questions and guidelines when devising therapeutic activities using these media:

1. How can the material be used in therapy with men?

2. What clients might appropriately view this material? For what clients, clinical diagnoses, or presenting problems would this material not be appropriate?

3. Pretend that a client was presented this material. What questions or issues would the client have about it?

4. Design follow-up activities for the material (e.g., discussion, paper-writing, drawing, drama).

5. Engage the client with introductory activities (e.g., asking questions to get a discussion going on the topic).

6. If the reading is to be conducted in the presence of the therapist, the therapist should participate in the reading, viewing, or listening phase. Ask leading questions and start short discussions throughout the reading.

7. Periodically, summarize what has occurred thus far (to be sure that "the message" does not get lost in the details).

8. Take a break or allow time for the client to reflect on the material.

Introduce some or all of these follow-up activities:

1. Retelling of the story.

2. In-depth discussion of the material (e.g., discussing right and wrong, morals, the law, strong and weak points of the main character).

3. Art activities (e.g., drawing map illustrating story events, creating a collage from magazine photos and headlines to illustrate events in the story, drawing pictures of events).

4. Creative writing (e.g., resolving the story in a different way, analyzing decisions of characters).

5. Drama (e.g., role playing, reconstructing the story with puppets made during art activity, enacting a trial for the characters).

6. Assist the patient in achieving closure through discussion and a listing of possible solutions or some other activity.

7. Avoid topics (e.g., abortion, drug use, crime) that might trouble the patient or family members, unless approved by the patient and concerned parties.

🖉 Exercise: Videotherapy

To illustrate the use of film we have selected three movies to discuss, with sample questions to explore. This same process can be used with other movies.

City Slickers

Healing themes: trying to find yourself, being stuck in a relationship, taking risks, father-son issues, commitment, effects of the past, parenting, friends, and support.

Main lessons:

- Good friends are an asset in dealing with the ups and downs of life.
- Lasting relationships require a heavy dose of commitment.
- The remedy for burnout is to do one's job well and have varied interests.
- Fathering is about doing positive activities together, as well as having long talks.
- Life is a series of "do-overs"—chances to try something once again, and to do it better this time.

Sample questions

1. What is the key message from the three friends regarding their fathers, and how would you relate these statements to your own father?
2. What was the role of Curly in the lives of the three leading men?
3. How did each of the men resolve their life changes and new approaches to life?

Field of Dreams

Healing themes: father-son relationship, reconciliation with the past, following one's dreams, heeding the voices within.

Main lessons:

- Never stop dreaming.
- Support for a partner means taking his or her visions seriously, even when they are not your own.
- Set goals and stick with them. Don't give up.
- To forgive a parent, it is necessary to walk in his or her shoes.
- Burnout may be a symptom of dwelling on mistakes.
- Sometimes one has to act on information that is less than complete.
- To reach your goals, help others reach theirs.

Sample questions

1. What is the place where dreams come true for each of the characters?
2. What reconciliation comes after the field is built? How will this give Ray greater peace?
3. Why will people come to the field of dreams?

The Great Santini

Healing themes: father-son relationship, alcohol abuse and its effects on the family, dominating personalities, masculine behavior, domestic violence, adolescent drinking.

Main lessons:

- Parents must protect their children from physical and emotional abuse.
- A spouse who is isolated needs a support system for reality testing.
- Fierceness and compassion can exist in a healthy mix.

- Assertiveness should be employed to break free from overbearing parents.
- Real men are strong enough to cry.

Sample questions

1. When you saw the basketball scene, what feelings and emotions were generated? Could you relate the scene to your experience with your father? Other men?
2. What are your reflections on the role of alcohol abuse in the family?
3. Have you dealt with dominating men like the movie's Bull Meechum? How?

Three: Art as a Therapeutic Tool

Art therapy uses the creation or viewing of art to help people discover and express their feelings. Unlike other forms of art appreciation, which may focus on the subject, form, or technique of the finished work, art therapy (which typically employs paint, clay, charcoal, pastels, or other art materials) focuses on the process of creation itself. Moreover, the activity is undertaken primarily for its healing benefits rather than for the creative end result; in fact, the piece of artwork may never be shown to anyone outside the therapy session. Once an image or representation has been placed onto a sheet of paper, molded from clay, or created in any of the other myriad ways that a work of art emerges, the creator then can relate to it and share its meaning with the therapist. That is therapy.

Art therapists believe that the act of making a piece of art triggers internal activity that contributes to physical, emotional, and spiritual healing. For people who are not able or ready to create art, going to an art museum or looking through art books can also be helpful. Simply viewing art refreshes the spirit and promotes relaxation.

While people have always expressed their feelings through art, art therapy as a profession has existed only since the 1930s. Among the fields that now frequently incorporate art therapy as part of the treatment process are clinical psychology (in which art is used to uncover hidden emotions) and physical therapy (which uses art to help build self-confidence and aid rehabilitation).

Child psychologists and family therapists often use art therapy because children have a hard time putting feelings into words. Art therapy has also become a vital part of the activities offered in many nursing homes, long-term care facilities, and hospices.

Art therapy helps healing in various ways. First, the aesthetic quality of the work produced can lift a person's mood, boost self-awareness, and improve self-esteem. Second, research shows that physiological functions, such as heart rate, blood pressure, and respiration, slow when people are deeply involved in an activity they enjoy. In addition, making art also provides an opportunity for people to exercise their eyes and hands, improve eye-hand coordination, and stimulate neurological pathways from the brain to the hands.

Because art therapy uses a language other than words, it is often employed in treating patients with physical or emotional illnesses who have difficulty talking about their fears and hopes or about their anger and other strong emotions. The creation of art helps people get in touch with thoughts and feelings that are often hidden from the conscious mind.

Art therapy is not only the careful and ethical facilitation of art-based directives, it is also the concern and respect that is given to the image and the emotional well-being of the maker. In regard to the respect that the image requires, an art therapist is careful not to interpret the meaning for the client so as not to let his own projection confuse or stifle the therapeutic value of the image. Some interpretation is inevitable, perhaps as a way to suggest general connections to previously mentioned material or to bridge the separation from awareness that the client may have about what he is now viewing. However, there are never times to be absolute about interpretation.

Health Benefits

The mere act of creating art has intrinsic benefits, according to art therapists. By promoting feelings of achievement, the creative process automatically boosts self-esteem and self-confidence.

Stress reduction is also a significant benefit. Repressing strong feelings can lead to a buildup of stress, and that stress can intensify pain as well as the symptoms of various diseases. Because art in therapy helps people access their unconscious mind and release pent up emotions, it has been found to be useful in treating those suffering from stress and stress-related ailments.

Art therapy is also used as treatment for behavioral problems and often serves as an ancillary treatment to psychotherapy. It is frequently part of inpatient psychological treatment programs, including those for substance abuse.

Patients recovering from trauma or serious injury often find art therapy particularly beneficial, as do people with chronic illnesses, such as Parkinson's or Alzheimer's disease. In addition to these uses, art therapy can also help people with a serious or terminal illness create a tangible record of their thoughts and emotions.

Art-making also has a healing effect, merely through allowing opposite brain activity to occur. This bypassing of intellectualization allows for the expulsion of emotions, giving visual representation to otherwise silent energies. In our society, much has been discussed about the intelligence capacity of individuals; however, little has been discussed about the creative intelligence that everyone possesses. In treatment settings, this "intelligence" is often overlooked in favor of didactic and psychoeducational forms of treatment. When the decision is made to provide an intellectual framework for recovery or therapy, coupled with emotional and nonverbal targeting, a fuller and enhanced form of healing can be reached.

The slightest mark on a blank sheet of paper can be considered a creative expression. Therefore, the client who has engaged in making such a statement has participated in the therapeutic domain.

The use of art therapy-based modalities in addiction and other treatment settings appears to be on the rise. Brian Blocker, MA, LMHC, who was consulted for this chapter, has been employed in primary addiction facilities as well as in those focused on aftercare and trauma, where art therapy was an integral part of the treatment team goals. In a treatment facility, art materials may be stark and basic; however, a pencil or pen and paper are generally sufficient. Colorful collages, beautiful and poignant masks, and enormous group painting projects adorn the walls of treatment centers all around the country. Display cabinets in waiting areas offer glimpses in molded clay of a man's pain or pure joy.

Art therapy is not an "adjunctive" form of therapy, although it often is regarded and referred to as such. Art therapy should not be utilized except by a licensed art therapist. The American Art Therapy Association (AATA) has specific requirements that a facility must adhere to in order use the term "art therapy" or "art therapist." In order to practice art therapy, the practitioner must meet the qualifications AATA has set forth, which require education and training through a graduate-level program from an accredited school. One generally must also meet state or national qualifications for licensure in order to practice as an art therapist. Further information about art therapy and art therapists can be found through the AATA website (http://www.arttherapy.org/) or by contacting the art therapy chapter for your state.

Four: Finding One's Inner, True Self: Poetry as Access to the Spirit

"Whatever you do or imagine,
  Begin it; be in your boldness.
  Being in your power has beauty
  And magic . . .
  It is why you are here . . .
  In life."

—Stephen Andrew

W hen working with men, remember this maxim: you sometimes have to hit them over the head with a hammer to get their attention, to get them to move from their left to right brains. One way of "hitting men over the head" is through poetry. The poet has a way of saying things that we mortals are unable to, what Emily Dickinson referred to when she described poetry as "that other thing." In Celtic mythology poetry is in the realm of *Tir na nÓg*, which is translated as "just the other side," just behind the thin veil of words.

So, we have found poetry to be a vital source of inspiration for men. We highly recommend poetry by David Whyte, who seems to speak especially to the male soul, as does William Butler Yeats, among many others.

We also recommend the following:

- *Crossing the Unknown Sea: Work as a Pilgrimage of Identity*, David Whyte
- "Anthem," "Hallelujah," Leonard Cohen
- *Snowbanks North of the House*, Robert Bly
- "Self-Portrait," "Sweet Ulysses," "Enough," "Revelations Must Be Terrible," "The Faces at Braga," "The Half Turn of Your Face," David Whyte
- "You, Darkness," Rainer Maria Rilke
- "Success," Ralph Waldo Emerson

There are many less famous but equally powerful poems specifically penned for and from the male perspective. Two of our favorite anthologies of such poems are *Men of Our Time: An Anthology of Male Poetry in Contemporary America*, edited by Fred Moramarco and Al Zolynas, and *The Rag and Bone Shop of the Heart: Poems for Men*, by Robert Bly, James Hillman, and Michael Meade.

Encouraging men to create their own poems can be powerful work. The depths to which a man will mine the gems of his emotional self, when given permission, are immeasurable. In his book *Writing from the Body*, John Lee details how a man might begin the process of awakening his writer's soul and quieting his inner critic. He offers many powerful exercises designed to help break through our mental, physical, and emotional barriers to writing.

Poetry can often help a man cut through his intellect and tap into a hidden part of himself that no one has ever seen. Encouraging men to write poems to a particular person or addressing a particular issue can have profound results.

The last use of poetry we will discuss here is group poetry. An interesting phenomenon occurs when a group of men offer what appear to be disconnected thoughts, without knowing the purpose. The following string of lines is the result of eight men, after completing a guided breath meditation with the directive to write down their vision, speaking aloud whatever sentence had come up for them to help them on their journey.

> Responsibility over fear.
> The world may be unpredictable, but stability will follow.
> Trust the unknown adventure.
> My feelings are the same, whether guiding or leading.
> Life is good, self as others, others as self.
> Uncertainty can be scary, or exciting and fun.
> Trust makes the difference.
> Care, power, self-reliance, superiority, ego.
> Let go, be at peace.
> However you choose to use it, poetry can be a
> powerful tool.

Five: Activities

"If we all did the things we are capable of doing, we
would literally astound ourselves."

—Thomas Edison

Adventure therapy is a type of experiential therapy that requires
people to work together in groups or that challenges an individual
to overcome a test and go beyond his normal comfort level. Activity
therapy of this nature addresses issues such as group and family dynamics,
problem-solving skills, communication, leadership styles, and support.
Programs such as Outward Bound, youth programs, correctional
programs, and corporate team-building have used adventure and
activity therapy for over forty years.

ROPES (Reality Oriented Physical Experience Services) and other
initiatives have been used in residential addiction treatment programs,

because these therapies "get to" issues that traditional talk therapy cannot, or that talk therapy gets to more slowly. Family secrets, control issues, fear, self-awareness, memories of past traumas, communication patterns, and issues of faith and trust frequently surface in adventure therapy.

ROPES has also been used in corporations, with volunteers, and with church and youth groups to achieve a variety of goals:

- Discover internal resources in the group

- Discover new skills and reduce stress within the group

- Motivate and revitalize

- Discover and build spirituality

When the subject of a ROPES course is brought up in conversation, many people visualize an obstacle course filled with various torturous and humiliating devices. For some people, the fear of the unknown is so great that they will go to almost any length to avoid experiencing a ROPES program. However, for those who take the risk and attend a ROPES day, their lives can be changed forever. The experience works by means of a "challenge-by-choice" philosophy, which lets the participants decide the extent to which they wish to participate in each activity. Within the first twenty minutes, fear fades as most people realize that ROPES is a different and fun way to learn how to work as a team by working through personal blockages. Success is determined by the group and is based on finding value in people's efforts.

Experiential learning models vary, but generally there are four distinct phases that comprise the learning cycle:

1. Experience
2. Reflection

3. Processing

4. Application back to experience

ROPES create a shared experience that sets the stage for learning. This experience allows the participant to look back and examine what he saw, felt, and thought during the event. The intent is to help participants understand what happened at a cognitive, affective, and behavioral level before, during, and after the activity. It is during this stage that the participant examines patterns of thoughts, feelings, and behaviors that occurred and tries to make links with similar occurrences in his life. Meanwhile, a certified ROPES facilitator can see and learn a great deal about the participants. Often, he will notice patterns of behavior and interactions of which neither the individuals nor their team are aware. As a result, the challenge becomes how to help participants become aware of their thoughts, feelings, and behavior and how to transfer this knowledge to their home, work, or school setting.

High ROPES courses (those that require significant installation fee and skilled trainers to manage) and other fixed low element challenges (those that may not be a high or challenging course but require a significant degree of challenge to the participant) can be expensive. There are portable challenge courses that cost far less than the construction of fixed platforms. Other low-cost activities are group jump rope, group juggling, minefield games, tug-of-war, hoop relay, rodeo throws, "traffic jam," and other games that involve little to no materials costs. By paying attention to props and simple things around the house and by thinking creatively, you can discover ways to develop your own adventure kit on a budget. Activities are powerful complements to traditional group work. Clients' stories are often revealed more swiftly through activities. Clinicians need training in the use of activities as they can be very powerful tools and need to be utilized appropriately. Activities are not parlor games to be used cavalierly. Rather, they need to be used skillfully and under close supervision and training. The following examples are feedback from two male ROPES course participants:

"As the day went on I thought nothing of my past and only thought of the present, which made me realize that I can't dwell on bad times. This is an important lesson for me as I move on with my life. I was also able to see the faces of my peers as I grabbed for their hands for help. It's getting easier to ask for help from other men and to face my fears."

"Today we learned how to trust each other. I learned perseverance and determination to not give up on things in front of me. I learned that reaching up and pulling myself up was like asking God to help me up, giving me the strength and courage to fight for my life. Reaching down to help someone else up was like using what God gave me to help them on their path. I also learned that if you fall or fail it's a lot easier to get back up with the support and encouragement of others."

For further information on ROPES course work, how to build one, where to get certified, and where to find one in your area, simply type the keywords "ROPES Courses" into your web browsing search engine.

Six: Questionnaires

As discussed throughout, men do well with concrete tasks, such as homework assignments and questionnaires. The following questionnaires were threaded throughout this book, and are reprinted here as one document for easier access.

Being a Man

1. What have you learned about men?

2. How would you complete these sentences:

- Men are

- Men usually

- Men never

- Boys are different than girls because they

- Boys lack

- Boys should be able to

- Boys won't want to

- Compared to girls, boys are more

- Compared to boys, girls are more

- Most of the men in my life have been

2. Think of a time in your life when a man came through for you, supported you. Who was that person? What did he provide? What do you take from that experience?

3. What are some of your expectations of women? (e.g., they put their needs aside in favor of men's, hide their intelligence, look to men to care for financial or physical tasks, are dependent on men, acquiesce to men's demands, take care of children, cook, clean house, defer to male authority, manage the feelings in a family or relationship.)

4. Which (if any) of these expectations were present in your family? What were you taught? What occurred in your family? Which of these expectations do you see your son or his friends adopting? Which do you find it hard to let go of as expectations for yourself?

5. How did you cope with the pressure to act like a man? When you were young did you feel you were tough enough? Did you try to act tougher?

6. Were you disrespected by adults for not acting like a man? What names were you called? Were you hit by your parents? By anyone else? What do you carry from these experiences?

7. What cultural, racial, or religious traditions do you identify with? What traditions do you value? What parts have lacked meaning for you? What traditions would you like to pass on to your sons?

8. How would you describe your spiritual life?

9. How would you describe your physical life? Do you feel tired, warm, etc.? Do you get enough sleep? Do you eat properly, exercise adequately?

10. What feelings of loss and grief do you have?

11. When you were a child, did your family use physical discipline?

12. What was the effect on you? Were you verbally mistreated, put down, teased, told you were stupid, or subjected to other negative comments? What were the effects of verbal abuse?

Turning Points in Your Life

Write your earliest memories of:

1. Your first day of school, first love, first kiss

2. Most recent illness

3. Your school years, especially high school

4. First job, first significant achievement, first sense of failure

5. Career changes

6. Marriage(s), children, births, weddings, life changes

7. First and most recent experience with death

Key Questions

1. Where do you want to be in five years (living, working)?

2. Describe the qualities of your relationships.

3. What activities give you meaning? Painful memories, experiences?

4. If someone were to give you a testimonial dinner, what would you want said about you?

5. How would you describe your purpose in living? Your place in the universe?

4. What gift would you give to your family today if all things were possible to give?

You and Your Father

1. Describe your father. What do you remember about him? What kind of person is/was he? What did he talk with you about? What didn't he talk about? How did he express his feelings? What feelings did he express? How did he relate to women, children, other men?

2. Complete this sentence: "What my father passed on to me was. . . ."

3. If your father was standing in front of you today, how would you complete this sentence: "Dad, I needed you to. . . ."

4. For what have you blamed your father? Your mother?

5. What other father figures were in your life growing up? Who were your heroes? What did you learn from them?

6. What qualities do you think are important in a father?

Work and Overwork

In your journal, write down all that apply:

- My family complains about my absence at evening meals because I am working late.

- I bring work home often.

- I have uncomfortable feelings about my strong work focus.

- At work I experience frustration about not seeming to ever get caught up.

- I often feel best when I am very busy, whether at work or home.

- I call in to work at least twice while on vacation.

- I postponed or changed my vacation dates at least once during the past five years.

- I have been quietly harboring a desire to work less and get off the work treadmill.

- I feel angry about all that my employer expects of me.

- Those close to me often express displeasure about my being away so much on business trips.

- I feel guilty when I leave work on time.

Answer the following questions.

1. What bothers me most about my current job and/or work climate?

2. If I imagine myself at the age of sixty-five reflecting on my life, what would have been important to me and what would not?

3. Have I shared my dissatisfaction about my current job situation with those I care about? If not, why not?

4. If I had more personal time available, what is one way I would spend it?

5. Can I downshift at work? What is stopping me from doing so?

6. What is most important in my life right now?

7. What is my greatest concern or fear about work?

8. If I created space for myself with respect to work, what would I do instead?

9. On average, how much time per week would I like to carve away from my work?

✎ Men and Money

1. Describe your current attitude about money. How important is it to you? Do you derive security from it? Do you use it to measure your self-worth? To measure your success? What does money mean to you?

2. Do you have a sense that you have enough money, assets? If not, how much more do you think you need to feel comfortable? To feel secure?

3. What would it mean to you to lose your assets? Your life savings? What would it mean to be poorer than you are?

4. What is your current practice with money, saving, spending, hoarding, self-indulgence?

5. Do you believe your current attitude and practices with respect to money enhance or detract from your spiritual life, your recovery?

6. How do you think you need to change your current attitude and practices with respect to money?

7. List your material possessions: cars, houses, stereos, computers, clothing, leisure- sporting equipment.

8. How do you feel about these assets and possessions? How important are they to you? What would it be like if you lost them? What would you least like to lose?

Men and Sex

1. Describe your current sex life. How do you feel about your sex life?

2. On a scale of one to ten, one being the worst sex life in the world and ten the best ever, how would you rate your current sex life? Why? Your past sex life? Why?

3. What is your current attitude about sexuality?

4. In what way do you believe your current sexual practices help/ hurt your emotional, physical, and spiritual well-being?

5. In what ways, if any, do you think you need to change your attitudes and practices about sex?

You and Your Partner(s)

1. Give a brief history of your personal, intimate relationships. Describe issues and concerns in these relationships.

2. What patterns have you noticed in your relationships? Were your relationships of short or long duration? Intense? Passionless? Passionate? Were you happy? What would you do differently now?

3. Do men around you avoid intimacy? How could you be more intimate? With whom? What ways do you avoid intimacy?

4. What would you gain by being closer to other men in your life?

5. List three things you'd like to tell another man. Are there things you don't know how to say, things about which you're embarrassed, ashamed?

6. Do you find it embarrassing to talk with men about personal

information? What specifically do you find embarrassing to talk about with other men?

7. Write the name of one man you'd like to be closer to. How can you make that happen?

8. Write the name of one man you love, one you have loved, one you care about, one who cares for you. These may be the same person or different men. Think of as many men as possible that fit the description.

Men and Their Children

1. How would you like to raise your boy(s)? To be connected to the environment? To express a variety of feelings? To take care of themselves physically and emotionally so they do not expect others to take care of them? To help others: the sick, poor, needy?

2. What kind of world do you want to create?

3. What do men stand for?

4. How different are boys and girls?

5. Make a list of what you consider to be male and female qualities.

6. Is there an age beyond which you find it hard to hug or hold boys? Why?

7. How do you withhold affection from older boys? Men?

8. Describe a time when you worried that your son or another boy wasn't tough enough.

9. How do you encourage boys to toughen up, suck up the pain, act like a man?

10. What kind of men do we need today?

11. Who are your "sons"? Boys to whom you act like a parent?

12. Which boys are hardest to see as your "sons"? Suburban, urban, rural, poor, well-off, disabled, gay, bisexual, African American, Asian, Latino, Jewish, Native American, White, immigrant, gang members?

13. Are you uncomfortable when your son comes home defeated, scared, having run from a fight? When he cries? Are you fully present to him then, or do you panic, withdraw from him?

14. Do you talk to your sons about personal matters? Do you listen to them?

15. In what ways have you assumed your sons or other boys you interact with are heterosexual?

16. When you were growing up, what were the messages given you about homosexuality? How old were you then? Where do you notice homophobia in the boys around you?

17. What do you love about your sons? What is unique about them? Positive qualities? Challenges they face?

18. Are there situations when you think it is okay to hit a child? To punish a child? To threaten a child? What do you gain/lose from threats, from hitting a child?

You and Children

1. To whom are you a father figure (biologically, socially, psychologically)?

2. Who are other youth to whom you might be a father figure?

3. If you have daughters, how can you support them? Sons?

4. How can you teach your sons to respect women, to treat women as equals?

5. What are ways you can teach children to be proud of their race, culture, religion, heritage, and to know about and respect the heritages of others?

6. How can you be a good model of tolerance and respect for youth?

7. When was the last time you told others/children that you loved them?

Helping Children

Answer yes or no to the following questions:

1. Do I love, acknowledge, and respect the youth in my life?

2. Do I tell them at least once a day that I love them?

3. Do I avoid blaming them for their mistakes?

4. Do I take out my anger, frustrations, past hurts, and disappointments on them?

5. Do I challenge them inappropriately?

6. Do I talk straightforwardly to them?

7. Do I help them heal their hurts?

8. Do I share power with them in an appropriate manner?

9. Do I help them work together and support each other?

Exercise: A Graph of Your Losses

Draw a timeline of your life. Include all the significant losses you have experienced. Date the losses. Write a sentence about what impact these losses have had on your life. What beliefs have you gained from each of these losses, either beliefs that constitute wisdom, or negative beliefs about your life?

Exercise: One Year to Live

Here's the bad news: you have been given one year to live. Here's the good news: you have unlimited resources to do whatever you wish to do. Question: what would you do?

Exercise: A Personal Creed

Stephen Covey, in his book *The 7 Habits of Highly Effective People*, speaks of the value of writing a personal mission statement, a creed in what you may believe. Write a personal creed. You may want to regularly review and update your creed.

Conclusion

In this book, we have sought to provide a pathway for men and women to explore what it means to be a man, or how you might live with the men in your life. We have provided practical tools to begin this journey of understanding manhood. There remains a paucity of literature geared toward men, and much of what is written addresses primarily issues related to aging or men's health. This book has sought to explore many of the key issues men face and can be a valuable asset to men, women, and care providers of men at various stages of life.

There is hope for a healthier, fully experienced male life. It must begin with rethinking and restructuring the male socialization process. Our collective wish is that those seeking to shift their experience may take some of the tools we have discussed and begin to fine-tune their own internal emotional machinery, and that their positive changes will be noticed and appreciated by others, who will then take on their own "re-creation." The possibilities are endless. We wish you much success.

Section IV Notes

1. Howard G. Rosenthal, "Homework Makes a Good Counseling Session Even Better," *Counselor Magazine*, July 2002, accessed at http://www.counselormagazine.com/columns-mainmenu-55/65-professional-development/440-homework-makes-a-good-counseling-session-even-bet.

2. Bernard Beitman, *The Structure of Individual Psychotherapy* (New York: Guilford Press, 1987).

3. Simon H. Budman and Alan S. Gurman, *Theory and Practice of Brief Therapy* (New York: Guilford Press, 2002).

4. Albert Bandura, *Principles of Behavior Modification* (New York: Holt, Rinehart and Winston, Inc., 1969).

5. Jay Haley, *Uncommon Therapy: The Psychiatric Techniques of Milton H. Erickson, M.D.* (New York: Norton, 1973).

Appendix I: Bibliography

The following is a bibliography of books recommended for assignment to clients, based on the client's diagnosis or presenting problem. It is not an exhaustive list. For further information on these books or other recommended texts for bibliotherapy, we refer you to the text by Michael Tompkins, *Using Homework in Psychotherapy*, and to Michael Gurian's user-friendly book, *What Stories Does My Son Need*.

Addiction and Recovery

The Addictive Personality, Craig Nakken

Children of Alcoholism, Judith Seixas and Geraldine Youcha

My Mama's Waltz, Eleanor Agnew and Sharon Robideaux

Perfect Daughters, Robert Ackerman

A Ghost in the Closet, Dale Mitchel

I'll Quit Tomorrow, Vernon Johnson

I Wish Daddy Didn't Drink So Much, Judith Vigna

Recovery: Plain and Simple, John Lee

Adoption

Being Adopted, David Brodzinsky and Marshall Schecter

The Primal Wound, Nancy Verrier

Shadow Mothers, Linda McKay

Let's Talk about It: Adoption, Fred Rogers

Aging

The Longevity Project, Howard Friedman and Leslie Martin

Alternative Medicine

Healing and the Mind, Bill Moyers

Healing Words, Larry Dossey

Healthy Aging, Andrew Weil

The Natural Mind, Andrew Weil

Anger

The Anger Workbook, Lorrainne Bilodeau

Angry All the Time, Ronald Potter-Efron

The Angry Teenager, William Carter

The Dance of Anger, Harriet Lerner

Facing the Fire: Experiencing and Expressing Anger Appropriately, John Lee

The Missing Peace: Solving the Anger Problem for Alcoholics, Addicts, and Those Who Love Them, John Lee

Attention Deficit Disorders and Other Behavior Problems

The Broken Cord, Michael Dorris

Driven to Distraction, Edward Hallowell

How to Handle a Hard to Handle Kid, C. Drew Edwards

Your Kid Has ADHD, Now What? Janette Schaub

Positive Parenting Your Teens, Karen Joslin

Real Boys, William Pollack

Behavioral Addiction

Codependent No More, Melody Beattie

Out of the Shadows, Patrick Carnes

Addiction & Grace, Gerald May

Cocaine Addiction, Arnold Washton

Chronic Illness

Alzheimer's Sourcebook for Caregivers, Frena Gray-Davidson

Coping with Alzheimer's, R. E. Markin

Cancer as a Turning Point, Lawrence LeShan

Conquering Pain, Ronald Prust and Susan Luzader

Facing & Fighting Fatigue, Benjamin Natelson

The AIDS Dictionary, Sarah Watstein and Karen Chandler

Creativity, Work, Stress at Work

The 7 Habits of Highly Effective People, Stephen Covey

Real Power, James Autry and Stephen Mitchell

The Web of Inclusion, Sally Helgesen

Crossing the Unknown Sea, David Whyte

Creating a Life Worth Living, Carol Lloyd

No More Blue Mondays, Robin Sheerer

Beat Stress Together, Wayne Sotile and Mary Sotile

Chained to the Desk, Bryan Robinson

Dealing with People You Can't Stand, Rick Brinkman and
Rick Kirschner

Difficult Relationships

Why Men Don't Listen and Women Can't Read Maps, Allan Pease and Barbara Pease

The Angry Marriage, Bonnie Maslin

Emotional Unavailability, Bryn Collins

He's Scared, She's Scared, Steven Canter and Julia Sokol

Too Good to Leave, Too Bad to Stay, Mira Kirshenbaum

After the Affair, Janis Spring and Michael Spring

Surviving an Affair, Willard Harley, Jr. and Jennifer Chalmers

Divorce

The Healing Journey Through Divorce, Phil Rich and Lita Schwartz

At Daddy's on Saturdays, Linda Girard and Judith Friedman,

Divorced But Still My Parents, Shirley Thomas

Do I Have a Daddy? Jeanne Lindsay and Cheryl Boeller

Helping Children Cope with Divorce, Edward Teyber

Mom's House, Dad's House, Isolina Ricci

The Essential Grandparent's Guide to Divorce, Lillian Carson

Exorcising Your Ex, Elizabeth Kuster

Domestic Violence

He Promised He'd Stop, Michael Groetsch

When Men Batter Women, Neil Jacobsen and John Gottman

The Courage to Heal, Ellen Bass and Laura Davis

Secret Survivors, E. Sue Blume

The Sexual Healing Journey, Wendy Maltz

Victims No More, Mike Lew

Grief and Loss

Men and Grief, Carol Staudacher

Grieving, T. Ranks

Giving Sorrow Words, Candy Lightner

The Healing Journey through Grief, Phil Rich

Necessary Losses, Judith Viorst

Saying Goodbye to Daddy, Judith Vigna

When Dinosaurs Die, Laurie Brown and Marc Brown

No Time for Goodbyes, Janice Lord

The Grieving Child, Helen Fitzgerald

A Broken Heart Still Beats: When Your Child Dies, Anne McCracken and Mary Semel

How to Survive the Loss of a Child, Catherine Sanders

On Children and Death, Elisabeth Kübler-Ross

Longing for Dad, Beth Erickson

Losing a Parent, Alexandra Kennedy

Motherless Daughters, Hope Edelman

When Parents Die, Edward Myers

Companion through the Darkness, Stephanie Ericcson

How to Survive the Loss of a Love, Melba Colgrove

Living with Loss, Ellen Stern

Widow to Widow, Genevieve Ginsburg

When Men Grieve, Elizabeth Levang

Intimacy and Sexuality

Couple Sexual Awareness, Barry McCarthy and Emily McCarthy

Is There Sex after Kids? Ellen Kriedman

Passionate Marriage, David Schnarch

The Soul of Sex, Thomas Moore

The Testosterone Syndrome, Eugene Shippen and William Fryer

LGBT Issues

Lesbian and Gay Parenting Handbook, April Martin

The Journey Out, Rachel Pollack and Cheryl Schwartz

Finding the Boyfriend Within, Brad Gooch

Intimacy Between Men, John Driggs and Stephen Finn

Coming out of Shame, Gershen Kaufman and Lev Raphael

Coming out Spiritually, Christian de la Huerta

Like Bread on the Seder Plate, Rebecca Alpert

The Other Side of the Closet: The Coming-Out Crisis for Straight Spouses, Amity Buxton

When Husbands Come Out of the Closet, Jean Gochros

Trans Liberation, Leslie Feinberg

True Selves: Understanding Transsexualism, Mildred Brown

Medications

Listening to Prozac, Peter Kramer

Beyond Ritalin, Stephen Garber and Marianne Garber

Straight Talk about Psychiatric Medications for Kids, Timothy Wilens

Men's Issues

What Is a Man? Walter Newell

The Man in Me: Versions of the Male Experience, Ross Firestone

Delusions of Gender, Cordelia Fine

Adam's Return: The Five Promises of Male Initiation, Richard Rohr

From Wild Man to Wise Man, Richard Rohr

Lonely at the Top: The High Cost of Men's Success, Thomas Joiner

Fire in the Belly, Sam Keen

Iron John, Robert Bly

Playing Life's Second Half: A Man's Guide for Turning Success into Significance, David Powell

The Irritable Male Syndrome, Jed Diamond

Stiffed, Susan Faludi

The Myth of Male Power, Warren Farrell

Male Menopause, Jed Diamond

Where Men Hide, James Twitchell

The Man Whisperer: Speaking your Man's Language to Bring out His Best, Rick Johnson

Our Mothers' Spirit, Bob Blauner

The Wild Man's Journey, Richard Rohr and Joseph Martos

Manliness, Harvey Mansfield

Money

Everything You Know about Money Is Wrong, Karen Ramsey

Financial Peace, Dave Ramsey

Overcoming Overspending, Olivia Mellan

Mood Disorders

The Anxiety Cure: An Eight-Step Program for Getting Well, Robert Dupont

If You Think You Have Panic Disorder, Robert Granet and Robert McNally

Moodswing, Ronald Fieve

The Childhood Depression Sourcebook, Jeffrey Miller

Winter Blues, Norman Rosenthal

Growing Up Sad, Leon Cytryn and Donald McKnew, Jr.

Breaking the Patterns of Depression, Michael Yapko

On the Edge of Darkness, Kathy Cronkite

Undoing Depression, Richard O'Connor

I Don't Want to Talk about It: Overcoming the Secret Legacy of Male Depression, Terrence Real

Obsessive-Compulsive Disorders

Passing for Normal, Amy Wilensky

Stop Obsessing! Edna Foa and Robert Wilson

Tormenting Thoughts, Ian Osborn

The Mindfulness Solution: Everyday Practices for Everyday Problems, Ronald Siegel

The Mindfulness and Acceptance Workbook for Anxiety: A Guide to Breaking Free from Anxiety, Phobias, and Worry Using Acceptance and Commitment Therapy, John Forsyth and Georg Eifert

The Mindful Way through Depression: Freeing Yourself from Chronic Unhappiness, Mark Williams, John Teasdale, Zindel Segal, and Jon Kabat-Zinn

Full Catastrophe Living: Using the Wisdom of Your Body and Mind to Face Stress, Pain, and Illness, Jon Kabat-Zinn

Parenting/Families

Bradshaw on the Family, John Bradshaw

Good Enough Mothers, Melinda Marshall

How to Talk So Kids Will Listen, Adele Faber

The Mother Dance, Harriet Lerner

The New Peoplemaking, Virginia Satir

Parents Do Make a Difference, Michele Borda

P.E.T. Parent Effectiveness Training, Thomas Gordon

The 7 Habits of Highly Effective Families, Stephen Covey

Touchpoints, T. Berry Brazelton

Mothers, Sons and Lovers, Michael Gurian

Schizophrenia

Is There No Place On Earth For Me? Susan Sheehan

The Quiet Room: A Journey Out of the Torment of Madness, Lori Schiller and Amanda Bennett

Schizophrenia: The Facts, Ming Tsuang

Spirituality

Awaken to Your Spiritual Self, Marie-Jeanne Abadie

Conversations with God, Neale Walsh

A Course in Miracles, Foundation for Inner Peace

Going to Pieces Without Falling Apart, Mark Epstein

Expect a Miracle, Dan Wakefield

The Road Less Traveled, M. Scott Peck

A Return to Love, Marianne Williamson

The Seat of the Soul, Gary Zukav

The Seven Spiritual Laws of Success, Deepak Chopra

The Spirituality of Imperfection, Ernest Kurtz and Katherine Ketcham

Tuesdays with Morrie, Mitch Albom

Working with Emotional Intelligence, Daniel Goleman

Step Parenting and Single Parenting

Blending Families, Elaine Shimberg

Family Rules, Jeannette Lofas

The Second Time Around, Louise Janda and Ellen Maccormack

The Single Father, Armin Brott

Suicide

Straight Talk about Death for Teens, Earl Grollman

Why Suicide? Eric Marcus

Verbal Abuse

Tongue Fu! Sam Horn

The Verbally Abuse Relationship, Patricia Evans

You Can't Say That to Me! Suzette Elgin

Appendix II: Videography

The following section is a listing of films and media that can be used in therapy, organized by topic and diagnostic category. As it is not the goal of this manual to provide a detailed analysis of each film and how it can be used in therapy, we refer you to Hesley and Hesley's *Rent Two Films and Let's Talk in the Morning* and Solomon's *Reel Therapy*.

For general inspiration, we recommend the following movies:

On Golden Pond

A River Runs Through It

Pay It Forward

Rudy

Field of Dreams

Billy Elliott

The Shawshank Redemption

It's a Wonderful Life

Strangers in Good Company

Shadowlands

Tender Mercies

About Schmidt

Million Dollar Baby

Tuesdays with Morrie

Babette's Feast

The Trip to Bountiful

Apollo 13

Patch Adams

A current all-time favorite movie about life, meaning, the purpose of existence, and quantum physics (now there's a combination) is *What the Bleep Do We Know!?* Not exactly romantic evening viewing, but certainly a thought-provoking and stimulating film that should engender significant discussion. There is even a study guide available on this film with questions and discussion points.

The following movies are excellent for portraying how support can be found from a number of sources, such as family, friends, colleagues, and assorted others who come in and out of our lives:

The Big Chill

Circle of Friends

City Slickers

Fried Green Tomatoes

Steel Magnolias

House of D

Peter's Friends

On the subject of men and women's search for meaning and significance in life, we highly recommend the following films:

American Beauty

The Apostle

Being There

Cider House Rules

Dead Poets Society

Short Cuts

Field of Dreams

It's a Wonderful Life

Jonathan Livingston Seagull

My Dinner with Andre

The Truman Show

There are many films demonstrating men's personal courage, without having to dip into the *Rambo* genre. Movies that portray courage, conviction, strength of character, commitment, and concern for others include the following:

Chariots of Fire

Master and Commander

Field of Dreams

The Pianist

Gandhi

Life Is Beautiful

The Shawshank Redemption

Forrest Gump

Video Work in Training and Supervising Counselors

Most films that are suitable for treatment purposes work well for training as well. Therefore, rather than repeat the recommended films for clients and counselors, the next section will discuss films by category for treatment, training, and clinical supervision. Also, it will be obvious that some films are applicable to a variety of categories.

The following is a list of films by diagnosis:

Narcissism: *All That Jazz*

Obsessive Compulsive Behavior: *As Good as It Gets*

Autism: *David's Mother*

Delusions: *Don Juan DeMarco*

Antisocial Behavior: *Falling Down*

Borderline Personality: *Fatal Attraction*

Depression: *Mr. & Mrs. Bridge*

Bipolar Disorder: *Mr. Jones*

Anxiety/Panic Disorders: *What About Bob?*

For addiction or substance abuse and dependence, we recommend the counselor and/or client view the following:

Soft Is the Heart of a Child (a wonderful, older film worthy of finding and adding to your or your agency's video library)

Afflicted

There are several important films that explore issues of diversity, discrimination, affirmative action, cultural mores, sexism and racism, gender equality, and civil rights, including:

A Star Is Born
Joy Luck Club
Philadelphia
A Raisin in the Sun
My Family
Rain Man

Regarding marriage, children, divorce, parental custody, family therapy, and parent-child relationships the list is lengthy and rich:

Kramer vs. Kramer
Ordinary People
Little Man Tate
Rudy
The Secret Garden
American Beauty
Mrs. Doubtfire
The Great Santini
To Kill a Mockingbird
Life Is Beautiful
Ma Vie en Rose
Mask
The Miracle Worker
Parenthood
Searching for Bobby Fischer

Many men we see will confront family and parenting issues, including concerns related to single parenting, blended families, sibling relationships, adoption, custody of children, letting go, family conflicts, and the empty-nest syndrome. Films are an excellent tool when working through such life issues. In these areas we recommend the following films:

The Accidental Tourist

As Good as It Gets

Mrs. Doubtfire

Tender Mercies

Ulee's Gold

Step Mom

Fly Away Home

Hannah and Her Sisters

Long Day's Journey into Night

Marvin's Room

On Golden Pond

Terms of Endearment

The Good Mother

Losing Isaiah

Breaking Away

Father of the Bride

Little Women

A River Runs Through It

For video work in couples and communication counseling and when addressing issues related to commitment in relationships, the following are appropriate:

The Doctor

Erin Brockovich

The Horse Whisperer

He Said, She Said

The Four Seasons

Husbands and Wives

The Postman

Scenes from a Marriage

When a Man Loves a Woman

About Last Night

The Age of Innocence

Groundhog Day

High Fidelity

Nine Months

An Officer and a Gentleman

The Story of Us

Films that address overcoming the pain and guilt of extramarital affairs, renewed intimacy, and dealing with divorce are:

Afterglow

Bridges of Madison County

Something to Talk About

Accidental Tourist

Pleasantville

Shakespeare in Love

Bye Bye Love
Kramer vs. Kramer
Starting Over
War of the Roses

The last film, *War of the Roses*, is an excellent example of the need for the therapist to be sensitive to the film's content and to whom she recommends the film, as the film is filled with violent images of conflict, resulting in the eventual deaths of the principal couple, portrayed by Michael Douglas and Kathleen Turner (now we've ruined the story for you). So, choose wisely!

For films dealing with conflict and negotiation, abandonment, premature death of a child, and widowhood, we recommend:

Strangers in Good Company

There are unique issues related to aging, death, and dying. The list of recommended films for these issues is extensive and rich:

Cocoon
On Golden Pond
Space Cowboys
Strangers in Good Company
My Life
Shadowlands
Message in a Bottle
Ordinary People
A River Runs Through It
The Son's Room

Movies about men and sexuality include:

About Schmidt

Ikiru

Something's Gotta Give

Movies about men and spirituality include:

Babette's Feast

Contact

The Doctor

Patch Adams

When clients are working through various psychopathologies, it is often helpful for them to see a dramatization of those pathologies, such as anxiety disorders and obsessive compulsive behavior. Outstanding examples are the funny and charming movies *As Good as It Gets* and *What About Bob? The Great Santini* is a dramatic portrayal of family violence and controlling behavior.

Other movies displaying psychopathology include:

What's Eating Gilbert Grape

Rain Man

Shine

Ordinary People

Suicide is dramatically seen in films including:

Dead Poets Society

Ordinary People

Whose Life Is It Anyway?

What's Eating Gilbert Grape?

Post Traumatic Stress Disorder (PTSD), phobias, and eating disorders are shown in:

Beloved

Saving Private Ryan

Fearless

The Truman Show

Vertigo

La Vie en Rose

Some counselors address issues related to teamwork and vocational concerns. We recommend the following movies:

Clockwatchers

About Schmidt

Field of Dreams

Patch Adams

Erin Brockovich

Good Will Hunting

Apollo 13

Top Gun

Movies about men and their fathers include:

City Slickers

Field of Dreams

The Great Santini

Swimming Upstream

Big Fish

Around the Bend

Movies about men and their children include:

Soft Is the Heart of a Child

Ordinary People

Movies about men and their addiction include:

Basketball Diaries

Days of Wine and Roses

The Lost Weekend

Addict (starring Johnny Depp, a film about methamphetami

Spun (also about methamphetamine addiction)

Born on the Fourth of July (starring Tom Cruise as Ron Kovic)

Requiem for a Dream

Owning Mahoney

The Gambler (about gambling addiction)

Love Liza (about sniffing gasoline)

When a Man Loves a Woman

Drunks

Tender Mercies (portrays someone in recovery from alcoholism)

Long Day's Journey Into Night by Eugene O'Neill (an excellent portr of a woman addicted to morphine, played by Katherine Hepbu

The following are films we recommend avoiding:

Arthur (glamorizes drinking and driving)

28 Days (sets group therapy in addiction treatment back a decade)

Harvey (where Jimmy Stewart plays a happy, comical drunk)

Up in Smoke (glamorizes drug use)

Easy Rider (glorifies hallucinogens)

Ray (although realistic, portrays a high-functioning Ray Charles on heroin)

When shown to professional staff, some films provide much fodder for ethical debate. *Final Analysis*, *Mr. Jones*, *The Butcher's Wife*, and *Prince of Tides* all show care providers sexually involved with their clients. On the other hand, films such as *Antwone Fisher*, *Ordinary People*, and *Good Will Hunting* raise interesting questions and ethical challenges for counselors and supervisors to consider.

When clients are working through various psychopathologies, it is often helpful for them to see a dramatization of those pathologies, such as anxiety disorders and obsessive compulsive behavior. Outstanding examples are the funny and charming movies *As Good as It Gets* and *What About Bob?* *The Great Santini* is a dramatic portrayal of family violence and controlling behavior.

Other movies displaying psychopathology include:

What's Eating Gilbert Grape
Rain Man
Shine
Ordinary People

Suicide is dramatically seen in films including:

Dead Poets Society
Ordinary People
Whose Life Is It Anyway?
What's Eating Gilbert Grape?

Post Traumatic Stress Disorder (PTSD), phobias, and eating disorders are shown in:

Beloved
Saving Private Ryan
Fearless
The Truman Show
Vertigo
La Vie en Rose

Some counselors address issues related to teamwork and vocational concerns. We recommend the following movies:

Clockwatchers

About Schmidt

Field of Dreams

Patch Adams

Erin Brockovich

Good Will Hunting

Apollo 13

Top Gun

Movies about men and their fathers include:

City Slickers

Field of Dreams

The Great Santini

Swimming Upstream

Big Fish

Around the Bend

Movies about men and their children include:

Soft Is the Heart of a Child

Ordinary People

Movies about men and their addiction include:

Basketball Diaries

Days of Wine and Roses

The Lost Weekend

Addict (starring Johnny Depp, a film about methamphetamine abuse)

Spun (also about methamphetamine addiction)

Born on the Fourth of July (starring Tom Cruise as Ron Kovic)

Requiem for a Dream

Owning Mahoney

The Gambler (about gambling addiction)

Love Liza (about sniffing gasoline)

When a Man Loves a Woman

Drunks

Tender Mercies (portrays someone in recovery from alcoholism)

Long Day's Journey Into Night by Eugene O'Neill (an excellent portrayal of a woman addicted to morphine, played by Katherine Hepburn)

The following are films we recommend avoiding:

Arthur (glamorizes drinking and driving)

28 Days (sets group therapy in addiction treatment back a decade)

Harvey (where Jimmy Stewart plays a happy, comical drunk)

Up in Smoke (glamorizes drug use)

Easy Rider (glorifies hallucinogens)

Ray (although realistic, portrays a high-functioning Ray Charles on heroin)

When shown to professional staff, some films provide much fodder for ethical debate. *Final Analysis*, *Mr. Jones*, *The Butcher's Wife*, and *Prince of Tides* all show care providers sexually involved with their clients. On the other hand, films such as *Antwone Fisher*, *Ordinary People*, and *Good Will Hunting* raise interesting questions and ethical challenges for counselors and supervisors to consider.

Movies about men and sexuality include:

About Schmidt

Ikiru

Something's Gotta Give

Movies about men and spirituality include:

Babette's Feast

Contact

The Doctor

Patch Adams